A Practical Book of

PRACTICAL PHARMACOLOGY - II

As Per PCI Regulations

THIRD YEAR B. PHARM.
Semester V

Dr. Hemant P. Suryawanshi
Assistant Professor,
PSGVPM's College of Pharmacy
Shahada.
Dist. Nandurbar.

Dr. Mukesh R. Patel
Assistant Registrar,
Shri. Govind Guru University
Gadukpur, Godhra, Gujarat

Dr. Sunil P. Pawar
Principal,
PSGVPM's College of Pharmacy
Shahada.
Dist. Nandurbar (MS)

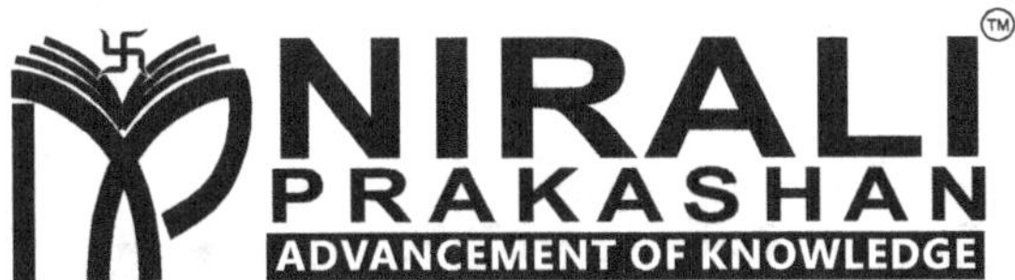

N3992

Practical Pharmacology - II   **ISBN 978-93-89533-99-6**

First Edition : **November 2019**

© : **Authors**

Published By :
NIRALI PRAKASHAN
Abhyudaya Pragati, 1312, Shivaji Nagar,
Off J.M. Road, PUNE – 411005
Tel - (020) 25512336/37/39, Fax - (020) 25511379
Email : niralipune@pragationline.com

➤ **DISTRIBUTION CENTRES**

PUNE

Nirali Prakashan : 119, Budhwar Peth, Jogeshwari Mandir Lane, Pune 411002, Maharashtra
(For orders within Pune)   Tel : (020) 2445 2044, Mobile : 9657703145
    Email : niralilocal@pragationline.com

Nirali Prakashan : S. No. 28/27, Dhayari, Near Asian College Pune 411041
(For orders outside Pune)   Tel : (020) 24690204 Fax : (020) 24690316; Mobile : 9657703143
    Email : bookorder@pragationline.com

MUMBAI

Nirali Prakashan : 385, S.V.P. Road, Rasdhara Co-op. Hsg. Society Ltd.,
    Girgaum, Mumbai 400004, Maharashtra; Mobile : 9320129587
    Tel : (022) 2385 6339 / 2386 9976, Fax : (022) 2386 9976
    Email : niralimumbai@pragationline.com

➤ **DISTRIBUTION BRANCHES**

JALGAON

Nirali Prakashan : 34, V. V. Golani Market, Navi Peth, Jalgaon 425001, Maharashtra,
    Tel : (0257) 222 0395, Mob : 94234 91860; Email : niralijalgaon@pragationline.com

KOLHAPUR

Nirali Prakashan : New Mahadvar Road, Kedar Plaza, 1st Floor Opp. IDBI Bank, Kolhapur 416 012
    Maharashtra. Mob : 9850046155; Email : niralikolhapur@pragationline.com

NAGPUR

Nirali Prakashan : Above Maratha Mandir, Shop No. 3, First Floor,
    Rani Jhanshi Square, Sitabuldi, Nagpur 440012, Maharashtra
    Tel : (0712) 254 7129; Email : niralinagpur@pragationline.com

DELHI

Nirali Prakashan : 4593/15, Basement, Agarwal Lane, Ansari Road, Daryaganj
    Near Times of India Building, New Delhi 110002 Mob : 08505972553
    Email : niralidelhi@pragationline.com

BENGALURU

Nirali Prakashan : Maitri Ground Floor, Jaya Apartments, No. 99, 6th Cross, 6th Main,
    Malleswaram, Bengaluru 560003, Karnataka; Mob : 9449043034
    Email: niralibangalore@pragationline.com

Other Branches : Hyderabad, Chennai

niralipune@pragationline.com | www.pragationline.com
Also find us on   www.facebook.com/niralibooks

Preface

Practical training is an important aspect of Experimental Pharmacology. This book is collection of specific methods used in understanding of basic principles of experimental pharmacology. In this an attempt has been made to highlight the practical areas of experimental pharmacology with intention to help students to learn basics in experimental pharmacology, various screening methods, their models and concept that provide advanced understanding of the subject. It provides a concise account of the preliminary methods and general principles which form the basis of pharmacological experimentation. We tried to achieve maximum coverage in the simplest way.

Practical book of Pharmacology-II is primarily aimed at the course requirements of the T. Y. B. Pharm. students according to PCI Regulations. It would also serve as a valuable resource of information to other healthcare science students. Some important features of the book are given below:

- Exactly as per the new syllabus prescribed by Pharmacy Council of India.

- Easy to follow, stepwise and self explanatory.

- Complete coverage to all topics.

- At the end of each experiment, short questions and answers along with MCQ's are given.

Practical book of Pharmacology-II is the outcome of numerous efforts of authors to assimilate the voluminous knowledge of experimental pharmacology.

Any suggestions for the improvement of this book are always welcome.

Authors

Syllabus

BP 507 P. PRACTICAL PHARMACOLOGY - II

1.   Introduction to in-vitro pharmacology and physiological salt solutions.

2.   Effect of drugs on isolated frog heart.

3.   Effect of drugs on blood pressure and heart rate of dog.

4.   Study of diuretic activity of drugs using rats/mice.

5.   DRC of acetylcholine using frog rectus abdominis muscle.

6.   Effect of physostigmine and atropine on DRC of acetylcholine using frog rectus abdominis muscle and rat ileum respectively.

7.   Bioassay of histamine using guinea pig ileum by matching method.

8.   Bioassay of oxytocin using rat uterine horn by interpolation method.

9.   Bioassay of serotonin using rat fundus strip by three point bioassay.

10. Bioassay of acetylcholine using rat ileum/colon by four point bioassay.

11. Determination of pA_2 value of prazosin using rat anococcygeus muscle (by Schilds plot method).

12. Determination of pD_2 value using guinea pig ileum.

13. Effect of spasmogens and spasmolytics using rabbit jejunum.

14. Anti-inflammatory activity of drugs using carrageenan induced paw-edema model.

15. Analgesic activity of drug using central and peripheral methods

***

Contents

***

Experiment No. 01

Aim: Introduction to *in-vitro* pharmacology and physiological salt solutions.

IN VITRO PHARMACOLOGY

In vitro pharmacology studies are done in the laboratory. *In vitro* pharmacology includes study of therapeutic effects of a drug in an isolated environment, such as cell lines or tissues. This setup conveniently eliminates whole organism's physiological influences allowing for a detailed analysis and a compounds impact.

In vitro pharmacological examinations, (for example, capacity of a medication to treat malignancy) are regularly first performed *in vitro* - either in a test tube or laboratory dish. A model would develop malignant growth cells in a dish outside of the body. This should be possible by utilizing various mediums which permit developing these cells free of the body.

Studies are normally done *in-vitro* first for ethical reasons. *In vitro* investigations enable a substance to be considered securely, as individuals or creatures are not exposed to the conceivable reactions or lethality of another medication. This learns however much as could reasonably be expected about a medication before presenting people to these potential impacts. In the event that a chemotherapeutic medication, for instance, does not chip away at malignancy cells developed in a dish, it is dishonest to have people utilize the medication and hazard the potential poisonous quality.

Advantages: *In vitro* pharmacological investigations are significant, in that they permit increasingly quick advancement of new medicines - numerous medications can be learned at once (and they can be contemplated in countless examples of cells) and just those that seem, by all accounts, to be strong go on to human examinations.

Disadvantage: A non-attendance of pharmacokinetics, in medicinal phrasing, is one of the critical downsides of *in vitro* pharmacological investigations. An absence of pharmacokinetics, just as a few different variables, can make it hard to extrapolate the outcomes to what may be normal when the medication is utilized in vivo.

PHYSIOLOGICAL SALT SOLUTIONS

Physiological salt solution can be defined as artificially prepared solution to keep isolated tissue alive under experimental conditions. They provide isotonicity, nutrition and act as a buffer when drugs are added. As animal experiments have to be done with isolated organs, it is necessary to use a certain number of physiological solutions of different ionic concentrations which almost act as a substitute to the tissue fluid.

It was "Ringer" who first introduced the idea that tissue could be kept alive by providing proper nutrition, oxygen, temperature, pH etc. The content of these solutions carries according to tissues and animals selected for experimentation. These solutions provide food material i.e. energy, oxygen, electrolytes like proportion as that present in tissue fluid. They exert same osmotic pressure as that of interstitial fluid i.e. isotonic with body fluids.

All PSS are prepared in distilled water. PSS are prepared fresh and utilized within 24 hours. Storage is not suggested because of microbial growth. While preparing the PSS, calcium chloride should be added last in the form of solution in order to prevent the precipitation of bicarbonate and isolated tissue will not live for extended period in cloudy PSS. Cloudy PSS also gives erratic response with drugs.

Any variant from the principle will lead to shrinkage or blotting depending on hypertonicity and loss of physiological function. For these two things should be remembered:

1. Prepare solution carefully with pure material.

2. They can be kept for about 24 hours and as they are good media for the growth of micro-organisms, they must be refrigerated and should be freshly prepared after 24 hours.

- **Following things should be carefully noted at the time of preparation of solution:**

    1. **Balance of ions:** Absolute quantity of each ion and preparation among each other especially with calcium and potassium must be maintained.

    2. **pH of solution/reaction of solution:** pH of various PSS varies from 7.3-7.8 depending upon organ. At lower pH value, tone of preparations tends to decrease and impact of medicament is also altered. pH affects tissue directly and by ionization. At elevated pH ionization is less and leads to alkalinity and thus improves cardiac and smooth muscle activity. During experiment there can be accumulation of metabolite which may change the pH. Buffering agents like HCO_3 and PO_4 are added in saline solution and solutions are changed frequently.

    3. **Glucose:** Introduced by "Locke" and serves as source of energy, increases contractility of tissue. Glucose is not essential constituent for amphibian's tissue, but essential for mammalian tissues.

    4. **Distilled Water:** Distilled water serves as a vehicle to dissolve various ingredients.

    5. **Control of temperature:** For consistent effect, it is important to maintain the temperature of PSS, particularly for mammalian tissue. For instance, when temperature of solution is below 37°C, tone of intestine is decreased, increased contracts become smaller and contraction and relaxation time increases; whereas amphibian tissues survive for longer time at normal environment.

    6. **Aeration:** Air, oxygen or oxygen + 5% carbon dioxide are required for the correct working of the tissues. Other than giving oxygen to the tissues, the flood of gas bubbles likewise blends the arrangements in the shower in this manner encouraging dissemination of the medications. The arrangement in the shower ought to be changed oftentimes in light of the fact that delayed air circulation will in general modify pH.

COMMON IONS USED IN PSS AND THEIR USES

1. **Sodium:** Responsible for maintenance of excitability, contractibility, rhythmicity of muscles and nerves.
2. **Potassium:** Responsible for increased relaxation of heart, increased neuromuscular transmission and excitability of nerves.
3. **Calcium:** Responsible for contraction of smooth muscle.
4. **Magnesium chloride and magnesium sulphate:** Responsible for relaxation of smooth muscles.
5. **Glucose:** Provides energy to the cell.
6. **Sodium bicarbonate:** Maintains the alkaline pH.
7. **Potassium dihydrogen phosphate or sodium dihydrogen phosphate:** Acts as a buffer.

DIFFERENT PSS AND THEIR USES

1. **Ringer Locke solution:** For isolated rabbit heart perfusion.
2. **Frog Ringer solution:** Used in rectus abdominis muscle, heart and other preparations of frog.
3. **Tyrode solution:** For experimentation in rabbit intestine and guinea pig ileum, rat ileum, etc.
4. **De-Jalon solution:** Used in rat uterus etc.
5. **Kreb's Henseleit solution:** For tracheal chain of guinea pig, vas deference, fundus strip of rat and aortic strip preparation of rabbit.

Table 1.1: Composition of Physiological Salt Solutions (PSS) (g/l)

Salts (g/l)	Ringer/ Ringer Locke	Frog Ringer	Tyrode	De Jalon	Kreb's-Henseleit	Mc Ewen	Hukovic
NaCl	9.00	6.5	8.0	9.0	6.9	6.6	6.6
KCl	0.42	0.14	0.2	0.42	0.35	0.42	0.34
CaCl$_2$	0.24	0.12	0.2	0.06	0.28	0.24	0.28
NaHCO$_3$	0.5	0.2	1.0	0.5	2.1	2.1	2.1
MgCl$_2$	-	-	0.1	-	-	-	-
MgSO$_4 \cdot$ 7H$_2$O	-	-	-	-	0.28	-	0.26
NaH$_2$PO$_4$	-	0.01	0.05	-	-	0.16	-
KH$_2$PO$_4$	-	-	-	-	0.16	-	0.15
Glucose	1.0	2	1.0	0.5	2.0	2.0	2.0
Sucrose	-	-	-	-	-	4.5	-
Aeration	O$_2$	Air	O$_2$/Air	O$_2$ + 5% CO$_2$	O$_2$ + 5% CO$_2$	O$_2$	Air

VIVA VOCE QUESTIONS

1. Define PSS.

Ans. Physiological Salt Solution can be defined as artificially prepared solution to keep isolated tissue alive under experimental conditions.

2. Enlist the various ingredients present in PSS.

Ans. NaCl, KCl, $CaCl_2$, $NaHCO_3$, $MgCl_2$, $MgSO_4 \cdot 7H_2O$, NaH_2PO_4, KH_2PO_4, Glucose and Sucrose.

3. Give the uses of various PSS.

Ans. **(i) Ringer Locke solution:** It is used in isolated rabbit heart perfusion.

(ii) Frog Ringer solution: Used in rectus abdominis muscle, heart and other preparations of frog.

(iii) Tyrode solution: For test of rabbit intestine and ileum of guinea pig, rat ileum etc.

(iv) De-Jalon solution: Used in rat uterus etc.

(v) Kreb's Henseleit solution: For tracheal chain preparations of guinea pig, vas deferens, fundus strips of rat and aortic strip preparation of rabbit.

4. Write significance of PSS.

Ans. As experiments in animals are performed with isolated organs, it's essential to utilize a certain number of physiological solutions of different ionic concentration which almost operate like a substitute to the tissue fluid. They provide isotonicity, nutrition as well as work like a buffer when drugs are added.

5. Define *In vitro* pharmacology with advantage and disadvantage.

Ans. ***In vitro* pharmacology** is the study finished in the laboratory and to study therapeutics outcome of a drug in an isolated environment, such as cell lines or tissues.

Advantages: *In vitro* pharmacological investigations are significant in that they permit increasingly quick advancement of new medicines - numerous medications can be learned at once (and they can be contemplated in countless examples of cells) and just those that seem, by all accounts, to be strong go on to human examinations.

Disadvantage: A non-attendance of pharmacokinetics, in medicinal phrasing, is one of the critical downsides of *in vitro* pharmacological investigations. An absence of pharmacokinetics, just as a few different variables, can make it hard to extrapolate the outcomes to what may be normal when the medication is utilized in vivo.

MULTIPLE CHOICE QUESTIONS (MCQ'S)

1. **PSS means :**
   - (a) Physiological Salt Solution
   - (b) Physiological Sugar Solution
   - (c) Both (a) and (b)
   - (d) None of these

2. **Role of Glucose in PSS :**
   - (a) Maintains the alkaline pH
   - (b) Acts as a buffer
   - (c) Provides energy to the cell
   - (d) All these

3. **While preparing the PSS, calcium chloride should be added last as a solution for prevention of precipitation of bicarbonate.**
   - (a) True
   - (b) False

4. **Tyrode solution contains ...... g/l of NaCl.**
   - (a) 6.0 g/l
   - (b) 6.6 g/l
   - (c) 8.0 g/l
   - (d) 9.0 g/l

5. **All PSS are prepared in distilled water.**
   - (a) True
   - (b) False

Answers :

1. (a)	2. (c)	3. (a)	4. (c)	5. (a)

****

Experiment No. 2

Aim: To study effect of drugs on isolated frog heart.

INTRODUCTION:

Frog:

Frogs are creatures of land and water, animals that occupy both land and water situations similarly effectively. There are believed to be around 5,000 unique types of frogs far and wide. Frogs are outstanding for their looped, sticky tongue which they anticipate out of their mouths to get creepy crawlies. Frogs are likewise notable for having the option to inhale through their skin just as their lungs.

Most types of frogs have projecting eyes, no tail, and solid and have webbed hands and feet, which help the frog in swimming, bouncing and notwithstanding climbing. Frogs tend to lay their eggs (known as frog bring forth) in lakes, however a few frogs have been known to likewise lay their eggs in enormous puddles. Infant frogs are called tadpoles and are totally water-based until the tadpoles create arms and legs and can move out of the water.

Most frogs eat creepy crawlies, other little arthropods, or worms, however various they additionally eat different frogs, rodents, and reptiles.

Frog heart:

Heart of frog is three chambered. It is dark red colored conical muscular organ situated mid-ventrally in the frontal fraction of the body cavity in between two lungs. The heart is enclosed in two membranes an inner epicardium and outer pericardium. The space between these two layers is called pericardial cavity in which pericardial fluid is present.

External structure of heart:

Remotely heart resembles a triangular structure. It is ruddy shading. It is 3 chambered other than sinus venosus and truncus arteriosus. Its foremost end is wide and back end is to some degree pointed. The front more extensive part is called auricles though the back part is called ventricles.

Auricles are two-chambered: left and right auricles. These auricles are separated remotely by extremely black out longitudinal interauricular groove. So it remotely seems one.

Ventricle is single chambered. It is funnel shaped fit as a fiddle with thick solid dividers.

Heart of frog consists of two additional chambers:

1. Sinus venosus

2. Truncus arteriosus

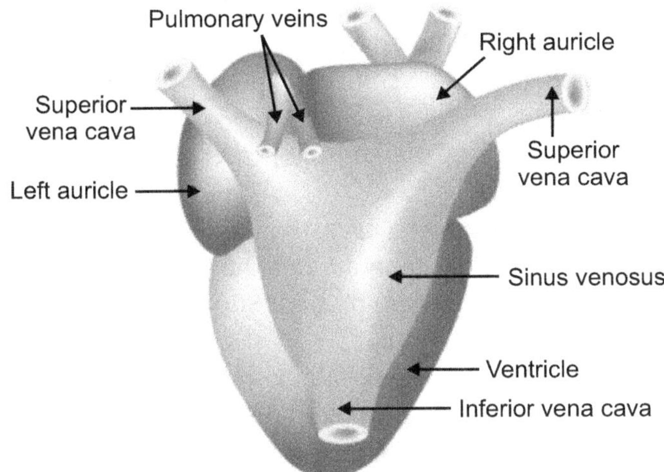

Fig. 2.1: Frog heart

Internal structure of heart of frog:

The ventral perspective on inward structure of heart appears two auricles, one ventricle, truncus arteriosus and the valves, to keep the blood streaming one way. The mass of heart comprises of three layers external epicardium, center mesocardium and inward endocardium.

Frog heart is 3-chambered with two auricles and one ventricle. The two auricles are isolated from one another by interauricular septum. Right auricle is bigger than left.

PRINCIPLE:

Heart is provided by ANS. Adrenaline goes about as an agonist. It follows up on beta receptors and builds pulse and plentifulness. Acetylcholine follows up on muscarinic receptors as an agonist and diminishes the pulse and abundance. Abundance convergence of potassium chloride stops the heart beat during diastolic stage. Overabundance centralization of calcium particle stops heart beat during systolic stage. Potassium and calcium particle follow up on cardiovascular muscle through non-receptor component of activity.

REQUIREMENTS:

Apparatus: Mariotte bottle, Syme's cannula clamp, recording drum, Starling heart lever, pin hook, thread, syringe and needle etc.

Drugs: Adrenaline (10 µg/ml and 100 µg/ml)

Acetylcholine (10 µg/ml and 100 µg/ml)

Potassium chloride (KCl – 10 mg/ml)

Calcium chloride ($CaCl_2$ – 10 mg/ml)

Distilled water

PSS: Frog ringer solution.

PROCEDURE:

1. Set up the assembly.
2. Sacrify the frog by pithing or by stunning.

3. Place the frog in a tray with ventral side facing up.
4. Make an incision to skin longitudinally and then expose the rectus muscle.
5. Make incision around the rectus muscle without damaging the frontal abdominal vein.
6. Expose the heart after cutting the sternum, then pericardial membrane remove and tie one part of aorta.
7. Put a knot around the inferior vena cava, then make a small cut for cannulation.
8. After cannulation with Syme's cannula, cut the other part of aorta and isolate the heart and perfuse with frog ringer solution. Supply frog ringer solution through the horizontal arm of the syme's cannula.
9. Place the heart clip on the heart apex, later connect it to a starling heart lever.
10. Record the normal heart beat on a smoked drum.
11. Inject 0.05 – 0.1 ml of adrenaline solution into syme's cannula. Immediately switch on the kymograph and record result of adrenaline for 2 minutes period. After 2 minutes turn off the kymograph till the heart beat and amplitude comes to normal.
12. Inject 0.05 – 0.1 ml of acetylcholine solution into syme's cannula. Immediately switch on the kymograph and record the outcome of acetylcholine (ACh) for 2 minutes period. After 2 minutes turn off the kymograph till the heart beat and amplitude comes to normal.
13. Administer 0.1 ml of KCl solution into syme's cannula. Immediately switch on the kymograph and record the result of KCl for 2 minutes period. After 2 minutes turn off the kymograph till the heart beat and amplitude comes to normal.
14. Inject 0.1 – 0.4 ml of calcium chloride solution into syme's cannula. Immediately switch on the kymograph and record the result of calcium chloride for 3 minutes period. After 3 minutes turn off the kymograph till the heart beat and amplitude comes to normal.
15. Observe the onset and duration of action of all, i.e. Adrenaline, acetylcholine, potassium chloride and calcium chloride.

OBSERVATIONS AND CONCLUSION:

1.   Adrenaline: It is responsible for increasing heart rate and amplitude. Heart contains beta receptors. Adrenaline stimulates beta receptors, thereby enhance the heart rate and amplitude. Drugs which block beta receptors (Propranolol, Atenolol etc.) are clinically used in hypertension and tachycardia.

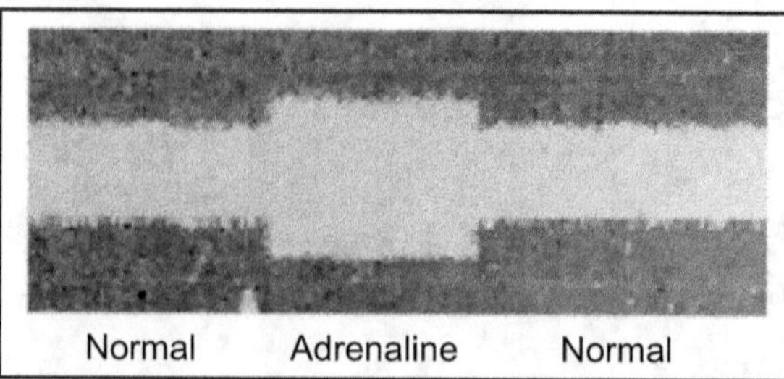

Fig. 2.2: Effect of Adrenaline on isolated frog heart

2.   Acetylcholine: It reduces the heart rate and amplitude. This effect is related to the effect produced by vagus nerve stimulation and it is via muscarinic receptors. Hence muscarinic blockers (Atropine, Belladonna extract) are responsible for reducing vagal tone and muscarinic actions.

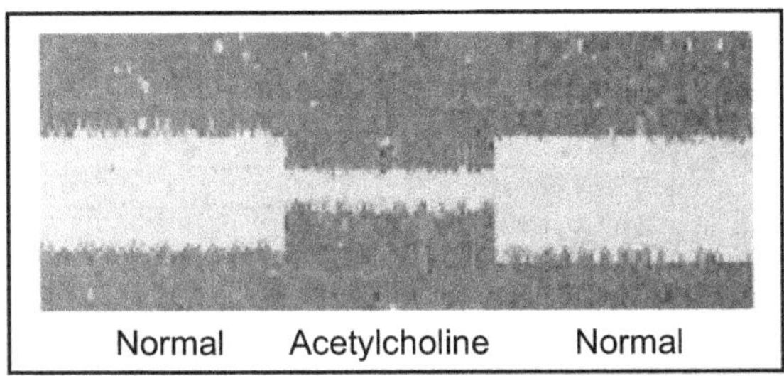

Fig. 2.3: Effect of Acetylcholine on isolated frog heart

3.   Potassium chloride in excess concentration: It reduces heart rate as well as amplitude.

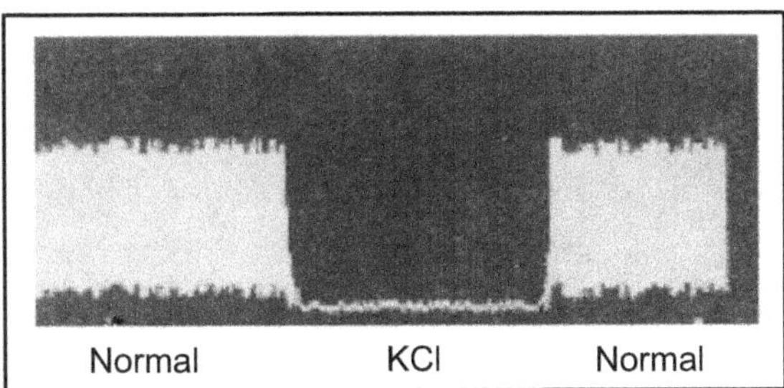

Fig. 2.4: Effect of KCl on isolated frog heart

4.   Calcium chloride in excess concentration: It stops beating of heart during systolic phase, an effect similar to digoxin poisoning. Calcium channel blockers like Verapamil, Diltiazem, Amlodipine etc., act as an antihypertensive agents.

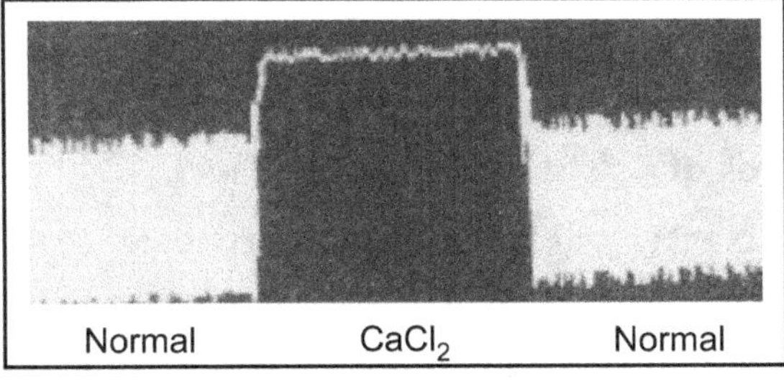

Fig. 2.5: Effect of CaCl$_2$ on isolated frog heart

Table 2.1: Effect of various drugs on isolated frog heart

Sr. No.	Drugs	Dose	Effect on isolated frog heart		
			Heart rate (beats/min)	Amplitude	Tone
1.	Adrenaline	10 µg/ml			
2.	Acetylcholine	10 µg/ml			
3	KCl	10 mg/ml			
4.	CaCl$_2$	10 mg/ml			

VIVA VOCE QUESTIONS

1. **Write action of adrenaline.**

Ans. Adrenaline increases heart rate and amplitude. Heart contains beta receptors. Adrenaline stimulates beta receptors and boost heart rate and amplitude.

2. **Give the principle of this experiment.**

Ans. Heart is provided by ANS. Adrenaline goes about as an agonist. It follows up on beta receptors and builds pulse and plentifulness. Acetylcholine follows up on muscarinic receptors as an agonist and diminishes the pulse and abundance. Abundance convergence of potassium chloride stops the heart beat during diastolic stage. Overabundance centralization of calcium particle stops heart beat during systolic stage. Potassium and calcium particles follow up on cardiovascular muscle through non-receptor component of activity.

3. **Give action of acetylcholine.**

Ans. Acetylcholine reduces the heart rate and amplitude. This effect is related to the effect produced by vagus nerve stimulation and it is via muscarinic receptors. Hence muscarinic blockers (Atropine, Belladonna extract) are responsible for reducing vagal tone and muscarinic actions.

4. **Write the examples of Calcium Channel Blockers.**

Ans. Calcium channel blockers like Verapamil, Diltiazem and Amlodipine etc. act as antihypertensive agents.

5. **Which animal and its heart has been utilized for this experimentation?**

Ans. Frog and heart of the frog is used for this experimentation.

MULTIPLE CHOICE QUESTIONS (MCQ'S)

1. **Select the correct dose of potassium chloride :**

   (a) 0.1 ml   (b) 0.2 ml

   (c) 0.3 ml   (d) 0.4 ml

2. **Potassium chloride responsible for :**

   (a) Boost HR and amplitude.   (b) Boost HR and decreased amplitude.

   (c) Decreased HR and amplitude.   (d) None of these

3. **Select the PSS exercise in this experiment :**

   (a) Tyrode solution   (b) Ringer solution

   (c) Frog ringer solution   (d) De Jalon solution

4. **$CaCl_2$ in excess does not stop the heart beating during systolic phase.**

   (a) True   (b) False

5. **Heart is supplied by ANS.**

   (a) True   (b) False

Answers :

1. (a)	2. (c)	3. (c)	4. (b)	5. (a)

***

Experiment No. 3

Aim: To study effect of drugs on blood pressure and heart rate of dog.

INTRODUCTION:

DOGS:

Dogs are widely used in biomedical research, testing, and education, particularly beagles, because they are gentle and easy to handle, and to allow for comparisons with historical data from beagles. They are used as models for human and veterinary diseases in cardiology, endocrinology, and bone and joint studies, research that tends to be highly invasive, according to the Humane Society of the United States. The most common use of dogs is in the safety assessment of new medicines for human or veterinary use as a second species following testing in rodents, in accordance with the regulations set out in the International Conference on Harmonisation of Technical Requirements for Registration of Pharmaceuticals for Human Use.

➤ **Normal values in dogs:**

1. **Blood Pressure:**

   Normal systolic blood vessel circulatory strain ranges from: 110-160 mm of mercury (Hg). Normal diastolic blood vessel circulatory strain ranges from: 60-90 mm of Hg. Normal MAP is in the range from 85-120 mm of Hg.

2. **Heart Rate:**

   The standard pulse in canines is 60-100 beats for every moment for enormous breeds, and 100-140 for little breeds. Bigger canines have more slow rates than little pooches, and mutts that are fit as a fiddle will have lower pulses than canines of comparative age and size that are not physically fit. Young doggies ordinarily have higher pulses; up to 180 beats for every moment is typical for canines as long as one year of age.

3. **Respiratory Rate:**

   Respiratory rate is the quantity of breaths every moment. Normal respiratory rates are evaluated when the pooch is resting. The standard respiratory rate for pooches is 10-34 breaths for each moment.

4. **Body Temperature:**

   All in all, pooches' body temperatures are higher than those of people. Truth be told, canine normal body temperature range is 100.5 – 102.5 F (38-39.2°C).

PRINCIPLE:

The blood vessel circulatory strain is characterized as the weight applied by the blood on the dividers of veins. Thus, Blood Pressure = Cardiac Output x Peripheral Resistance. The heart and veins are under the influence of autonomic sensory system. Both thoughtful and parasympathetic nerves supply the heart.

In general sympathetic stimulation (administration of adrenaline or noradrenaline) increases the CO as well as resistance to the flow leading to an increased blood pressure.

Alternatively, parasympathetic stimulation (administration of acetylcholine) decreases cardiac output which lowers the blood pressure. Drugs which increase blood pressure are called pressor agents and those which decrease are called depressor agents.

REQUIREMENTS:

Animal: Dog

Apparatus: Dog operating table, Kymograph, arterial cannula, venous cannula, tracheal cannula, 'U' shaped or Poiseuille's mercury manometer, connecting rubber tubing, dissecting instruments, syringes and threads, ECG machine etc.

Anesthetic agent: Pentobarbitone sodium (45 mg/kg, IV, stock solution - 45 mg/ml of the drug, administer 1 ml/kg of body weight).

Drugs and solutions:

Sodium citrate (8.5%) anticoagulant

Saline (0.9% NaCl)

Adrenaline (100 µg/ml)

Noradrenaline (100 µg/ml)

Isoprenaline (100 µg/ml)

Acetylcholine (100 µg/ml)

PROCEDURE:

1. An adult healthy dog is weighed and pentobarbitone sodium is administered to produce anesthesia (45 mg/kg given intravenously).
2. The animal is laid down on the operation table and its limbs are tied. From femoral triangle femoral vein is dissected and it is cannulated with thin polythene tube, linked to three way cannula. This is to administer various drugs and solutions.
3. Trachea and two carotid arteries expose by making an incision in the neck. Now the tracheal cannula is placed into the trachea. This is to record result of drug substances on respiration and to provide artificial respiration, if necessary.
4. The arterial cannula is cannulated in one carotid artery and it is joined to the 'U' Poiseuille's manometer. The gap between manometer and the arterial cannula is filled with sodium citrate and care is taken to avoid entry of any air bubble.
5. Record the base line means blood pressure response in addition to record the heart rate.
6. Various drugs are administered through femoral venous cannula and outcome is recorded. Usually the agonists be administered in the quantity of 2-10 µg/kg whereas, antagonists are administered with the quantity of 2 mg/kg. Antagonists are given in diluted form, to avoid any direct effect.

7. Note the sequence of result (response) i.e. increase in BP, heart rate, the vagal notch, BP declining below the base line and recovery to pre drug base line.
8. Wait for 5-10 minutes. Give sufficient gap (5-10 minutes) between outcomes of two drugs.
9. Now heart rate is recorded by Lead ECG.
10. Record normal BP and HR.

OBSERVATION AND DISCUSSION:

Adrenaline:

Adrenaline is a sympathomimetic catecholamine which produces effect through alpha, $Beta_1$ and $Beta_2$ receptors. Because of $Beta_1$ receptor stimulation, there is rapid boost in HR and power of contraction. Immediately due to reflex inhibition, there is slight decrease; but drug reaches the periphery where $Alpha_1$ receptor stimulation produces vasoconstriction and hence, more increase in BP is noted. Notch is seen due to sudden changes in response.

Adrenaline action is slowly terminated by uptake of monoamine oxidase (MAO) and catechol-o-methyl transferences (COMT). When level of adrenaline is reduced, $Beta_2$ receptors action predominates and because of that slight reduction in BP (secondary fall) is seen.

Noradrenaline:

Noradrenaline is a sympathomimetic catecholamine having predominantly alpha receptor action. The impact of NA differs from that of adrenaline that HR is not increased. Only increase in BP is seen and this is because of vasoconstriction of blood vessels specially those which supply blood to skin and mucosa. Since beta action of NA is not seen, the impact of rise in BP is more than adrenaline only.

Isoprenaline:

It is a sympathomimetic amine which produces explicit $Beta_1$ and $Beta_2$ receptor agonistic activity. $Beta_1$ receptors present in heart are energized by isoprenaline because of which there is increment in pulse and pulse. Medication arrives at outskirts there happens vasodilation of veins uncommonly which are provided to skeletal muscle. Because of this there is fall in pulse.

Isoprenaline isn't the substrate for take-up, henceforth, the end of move makes time and there is postponed recuperation.

Acetylcholine:

It is a parasympathomimetic specialist which can invigorate both muscarinic just as nicotinic receptors. Be that as it may, in low dosages it delivers just muscarinic receptor activity and henceforth, there is fall in pulse because of widening of veins.

The activity of Acetylcholine (ACh) is quickly ended by cholinesterase catalyst and consequently, the reaction of Acetylcholine (ACh) gets immediately recuperated. Pulse does not change because of Acetylcholine (ACh).

OBSERVATIONS:

Table 3.1: Effect of various drugs on blood pressure and heart rate of dog

Sr. No.	Drugs	Dose	Effect on	
			Blood Pressure (mm Hg)	**Heart rate (beats/min.)**
1.	Saline	-		
2.	Adrenaline	100 µg/ml		
3	Noradrenaline	100 µg/ml		
4.	Isoprenaline	100 µg/ml		
5.	Acetylcholine	100 µg/ml		

VIVA VOCE QUESTIONS

1. **What is normal blood pressure in dogs?**

Ans. Normal systolic blood vessel circulatory strain in dogs ranges from: 110-160 mm of mercury (Hg). Normal diastolic blood vessel circulatory strain ranges from: 60-90 mm of Hg. Normal MAP is in the range from 85-120 mm of Hg.

2. **Define heart rate and give its normal value in dogs.**

Ans. The standard pulse in canines is 60-100 beats for every moment for enormous breeds, and 100-140 for little breeds. Bigger canines have more slow rates than little pooches, and mutts that are fit as a fiddle will have lower pulses than canines of comparative age and size that are not physically fit. Young doggies ordinarily have higher pulses; up to 180 beats for every moment is typical for canines as long as one year of age.

3. **Explain action of adrenaline on dog heart.**

Ans. Adrenaline is a sympathomimetic catecholamine which produces effect through Alpha, $Beta_1$ and $Beta_2$ receptors. Because of $Beta_1$ receptor stimulation there is rapid boost in HR and power of contraction. Immediately due to reflex inhibition there is slight decrease, but drug reaches the periphery where $Alpha_1$ receptor stimulation produces vasoconstriction and hence, more increase in BP is noted. Notch is seen due to sudden changes in response.

Adrenaline action is slowly terminated by uptake of monoamine oxidase (MAO) and catechol-o-methyl transferences (COMT). When level of adrenaline is reduced, $Beta_2$ receptors action predominates and because of that slight reduction in BP (secondary fall) is seen.

4. **Give the principle in dog heart experiment.**

Ans. The blood vessel circulatory strain is characterized as the weight applied by the blood on the dividers of veins. Thus, Blood Pressure = Cardiac Output × Peripheral Resistance. The heart and veins are under the influence of autonomic sensory system. Both thoughtful and parasympathetic nerves supply the heart.

In general sympathetic stimulation (administration of adrenaline or noradrenaline) increases the CO as well as resistance to the flow leading to an increased blood pressure.

Alternatively, parasympathetic stimulation (administration of acetylcholine) decreases cardiac output which lowers the blood pressure. Drugs which increase blood pressure are called pressor agents and those decrease are called depressor agents.

5. Explain the effect of isoprenaline on dog heart.

Ans. It is a sympathomimetic amine which produces explicit $Beta_1$ and $Beta_2$ receptor agonistic activity. $Beta_1$ receptors present in heart are energized by isoprenaline because of which there is increment in pulse. Medication arrives at outskirts there happens vasodilation of veins uncommonly which are provided to skeletal muscle. Because of this there is fall in pulse.

Isoprenaline isn't the substrate for take-up, henceforth, the end of move makes time and there is postponed recuperation.

MULTIPLE CHOICE QUESTIONS (MCQ'S)

1. **Select the amount of Pentobarbitone sodium :**
   (a) 35 mg/kg
   (b) 40 mg/kg
   (c) 45 mg/kg
   (d) 50 mg/kg

2. **Action of Ach on dog heart via muscarinic receptors :**
   (a) Increase in BP
   (b) Fall in BP
   (c) No change in BP
   (d) None of these

3. **Select normal body temperature in dogs.**
   (a) 35-36.2°C
   (b) 36-37.2°C
   (c) 37-38.2°C
   (d) 38-39.2°C

4. **Heart is supplied by both sympathetic and parasympathetic nerve.**
   (a) True
   (b) False

5. **Isoprenaline is responsible for stimulation of $Beta_1$, due to that there is rise in BP and HR.**
   (a) True
   (b) False

Answers:

1. (c)	2. (b)	3. (d)	4. (a)	5. (a)

***

Experiment No. 4

Aim: To study diuretic activity of drugs using rat/mice.

INTRODUCTION:

DIURETICS:

A diuretic is any substance that increases the production of urine. Diuretics are used in treatment of various diseases like Cardiac failure, liver cirrhosis, hypertension, water poisoning, and certain kidney diseases etc.

➤ **Classification of Diuretics:**
1. **Loop diuretics:** Furosemide, ethacrynic acid and torsemide.
2. **Thiazide-type diuretics:** Hydrochlorothiazide.
3. **Carbonic anhydrase inhibitors:** Acetazolamide and methazolamide.
4. **Potassium Sparing Diuretics:**
    (a) Aldosterone antagonists: Spironolactone, eplerenone and potassium canreonate.
    (b) Sodium channel blockers: Amiloride and Triamterene.
5. **Osmotic Diuretics:** Mannitol

➤ **Loop Diuretics:**

Loop diuretics will be diuretics that demonstrate at the rising loops of Henle in the kidney. They are principally utilized in medication to treat hypertension and edema regularly because of congestive heart disappointment or renal deficiency.

Mechanism of Action: Loop diuretics follow up on the $Na^+/K^+/2Cl^-$ symporter (cotransporter) in the thick rising appendage of the loop of Henle to restrain sodium and chloride reabsorption. This is accomplished by seeking the Cl-restricting site. Since magnesium and calcium reabsorption in the thick climbing appendage is subject to the positive lumen voltage angle set up by potassium reusing through renal external medullary potassium channel, circle diuretics additionally restrain their reabsorption. By disturbing the reabsorption of these particles, loop diuretics avoid the age of a hypertonic renal medulla. Without such a concentrated medulla, water has less of an osmotic main impetus to leave the gathering pipe framework, at last bringing about expanded urine production. Loop diuretics cause a reduction in the renal blood stream by this component. This diuresis leaves less water to be reabsorbed into the blood, bringing about a reduction in blood volume.

The aggregate impacts of diminished blood volume and vasodilation decline circulatory strain and improve edema.

Clinical Indication: Loop diuretics are essentially utilized in the accompanying signs:

- Edema related with heart disappointment, hepatic cirrhosis, renal hindrance, nephrotic disorder.

- Hypertension.

- Adjunct in cerebral edema where quick diuresis is required (IV infusion).

They are likewise at times utilized in the administration of extreme hypercalcemia in blend with satisfactory rehydration.

Adverse Effects: ADRs include: Hyponatremia, hypokalemia, hypomagnesaemia, dehydration, hyperuricemia, gout, dizziness, postural hypotension and syncope etc.

REQUIREMENTS:

Equipments and Apparatus: Metabolic cages, graduated measuring cylinder, oral dosing tube etc.

Animal: Rat/Mice

Drugs and Solutions: Normal saline (0.9%), Urea (900 mg/kg; oral), Hydroflumethiazide (1 mg/kg; oral), Furosemide (5 mg/kg; oral).

PRINCIPLE:

Diuretics are the compounds which build stream of urine. Ordinary urine yield in rodents is little (1-2 ml/rodent/day). Subsequently to get the quantifiable amount the rats/mice are first hydrated. The urine yield is expanded after organization of diuretics like urea, hydroflumethiazide and furosemide. Increment in volume of urine is estimated with the assistance of measuring cylinder and compare with normal urine yield.

PROCEDURE:

1. Albino rats (150 - 200 g) are fasted (deprived of food and water) overnight and saline (25 ml/kg) is administered orally by using oral feeding cannula.
2. These animals are divided into four groups containing three rats in each as follows :
   (a) First group - only normal saline.
   (b) Second group - Saline + Urea (900 mg/kg; oral)
   (c) Third group - Saline + Hydroflumethiazide (1 mg/kg; oral)
   (d) Fourth group - Saline + Furosemide (5 mg/kg; oral)
3. Following the drug administration, animals are kept in the four different metabolic cages.
4. Measuring cylinder is used for collection of urine.
5. Time, when the first drop of urine is collected in a cylinder for each group is noted and the volume is recorded at intervals of 15 minutes for 3 - 4 hours.
6. The difference in the volume collected at different time intervals and total volume can be compared with various diuretics.

OBSERVATIONS AND DISCUSSION:

Table 4.1: Effect of drugs on urine output in rats/mice

	Groups	1	2	3	4
Amount of urine collected (ml)	After 15 minutes				
	After 30 minutes				
	After 1 hour				
	Total Volume				

➢ **Metabolic cage:**

Metabolic cages give an ideal separation of dejection and water through the special style of the funnel and of the separation cone. Accommodating mice or rats, metabolic cages supply 99% separation potency of water and dejection, reassuring most purity of samples. Animal waste is directed through a group funnel and onto a linear diffuser. The diffuser permits solid come to travel down the highest ridges of a 50 % incline, passing over a water port, and into a faecal assortment vessel. Liquid waste flows on grooves down the inclined diffuser, passing through the water port, and into a water assortment vessel. A water device prevents excess water from splashing and contaminating faecal specimen. Separate water and dejection samples area unit collected in 2 common place 50 ml centrifuge vessel.

VIVA VOCE QUESTIONS

1. **Define Diuretics and write its uses.**

Ans. A diuretic is any substance that increases the production of urine. Diuretics are used in treatment of various diseases like Cardiac failure, liver cirrhosis, hypertension, water poisoning, and certain kidney diseases etc.

2. **Classify diuretics with examples.**

Ans. (a) **Loop diuretics:** Furosemide, Ethacrynic acid and Torsemide.

  (b) **Thiazide-type diuretics:** Hydrochlorothiazide.

  (c) **Carbonic anhydrase inhibitors:** Acetazolamide and Methazolamide.

  (d) **Osmotic diuretics:** Mannitol.

3. **Write adverse effects of diuretics.**

Ans. Adverse effects of diuretics include hyponatremia, hypokalemia, hypomagnesaemia, dehydration, hyperuricemia, gout, dizziness, postural hypotension, syncope etc.

4. **Give MOA of loop diuretics.**

Ans. Loop diuretics follow up on the $Na^+/K^+/2Cl^-$ symporter (cotransporter) in the thick rising appendage of the loop of Henle to restrain sodium and chloride reabsorption. This is accomplished by seeking the Cl-restricting site. Since magnesium and calcium reabsorption in the thick climbing appendage is subject to the positive lumen voltage angle set up by potassium reusing through renal external medullary potassium channel, circle diuretics additionally restrain their reabsorption. By disturbing the reabsorption of these particles, loop diuretics avoid the age of a hypertonic renal medulla. Without such a concentrated medulla, water has less of an osmotic main impetus to leave the gathering pipe framework, at last bringing about expanded urine production. Loop diuretics cause a reduction in the renal blood stream by this component. This diuresis leaves less water to be reabsorbed into the blood, bringing about a reduction in blood volume.

5. Give the uses of loop diuretics.

Ans. • Edema related with heart disappointment, hepatic cirrhosis, renal hindrance, nephrotic disorder.

    • Hypertension.

    • Adjunct in cerebral edema where quick diuresis is required (IV infusion).

    They are also sometimes used in the management of severe hypercalcemia in combination with adequate rehydration.

MULTIPLE CHOICE QUESTIONS (MCQ'S)

1. Select the example of osmotic diuretics :

  (a) Furosemide   (b) Mannitol

  (c) Amiloride   (d) Acetazolamide

2. Loop diuretic agents are used in :

  (a) Edema   (b) Hypertension

  (c) Hypercalcemia   (d) All of these

3. Diuretics are responsible for :

  (a) Increase in urine output   (b) Decrease in urine output

  (c) Normal urine output   (d) All of these

4. Select the normal urine output range in rats :

  (a) 2 - 4 ml/rat/day   (b) 3 - 4 ml/rat/day

  (c) 1 - 2 ml/rat/day   (d) 4 - 5 ml/rat/day

5. Loop diuretics act on the $Na^+/K^+/2Cl^-$ present in ascending limb.

  (a) True   (b) False

Answers:

1. (b)	2. (d)	3. (a)	4. (c)	5. (a)

✱✱✱

Experiment No. 5

Aim: To study Dose Response Curve (DRC) of acetylcholine using frog rectus abdominis muscle.

INTRODUCTION:

Dose response curve (DRC) demonstrates hierarchical responses to medication or agonists wherever a rise in response is recorded with a later increase within the dose or the concentration of the drug. The DRC is sigmoid or S – formed. The primary half (25% graph) of the curve has poor discrimination between the doses, whereas the center portion of the curve shows bigger sensitivity to completely different concentrations and therefore the responses to increasing concentration square measure linearly differentiated. The last part of the curve (plateau) shows the ceiling result wherever no additional increase within the response is seen with more increase within the dose. The additive DRC obtained by increasing the concentration of the drug within the organ tub step by step while not laundry the preceding doses. This method is easy and fewer time overwhelming. It's usually used in those preparations wherever the tissue is slowly getting and slowly restful, but this technique is not fitted to the medication that show fade development. When the doses square measure enlarged in patterned advance (logarithmic intervals) and therefore the response is plotted against logarithms of doses, the link is termed dose response curve.

The logarithmic transformation of doses offer some advantages such as

1. The linear portion of the sigmoid curve becomes more straight.
2. Comparison of two DRC is much simpler.
3. Large dose range can be plotted which is otherwise difficult in DRC.
4. The error is distributed all through the graph, free of the dose.

The study of concentration or DRC curve indicates

1. Relative potency of the medicine or agonist. The drug is more potent when the curve is more towards the left and the vice versa.
2. Error and reliability (accuracy) of the bioassay is indicated by slope of the curve. Steeper the slope, precise is the assay and vice versa.

PRINCIPLE:

Frog rectus abdominis muscle is a voluntary muscle. At the neuromuscular junction, a nerve impulse liberates acetylcholine from the nerve ending into the cleft between nerve fiber as well as muscle. This acetylcholine causes a depolarization of the muscle fiber which in turns sets off a muscle action potential, and contraction of the muscle fiber. The muscle fibers of lower species like frog are multiple innervated and hence nerve stimulation causes persistent depolarization and a prolonged slow contraction of muscle. Local administration of acetylcholine also produces similar effect. Frog rectus abdominis muscle contains nicotinic (N_2) receptors. Acetylcholine work as an agonist.

REQUIREMENTS:

Equipments and Apparatus: Rotating drum, student organ bath, aerator, frontal writing lever, haemostatic forceps, mariotte bottle, tuberculine syringe, etc.

Animal: Frog.

Tissue: Rectus abdominis muscle.

Drug: Acetylcholine (Stock solution –1 mg/ml)

PSS: Frog Ringer solution.

Tension on the tissue: 1 gm.

Magnification: 5-7 times.

PROCEDURE:

1. Set up the assembly.
2. Pith a frog by passing a needle through the occipito-atlantic junction between brains with the spinal cord. The stretching of the limbs indicates that the pithing is proper.
3. Place the frog in a tray with the ventral side facing up.
4. Pick up the skin of abdomen by using forceps and make proper cut to open the abdomen.
5. Cut along the margin of the rectus abdominis muscle, and then make an incision throughout the sternum just above the base.
6. Separate the anterior abdominal vein and rectus abdominis muscle.
7. Lift the muscle gently and divide the muscle longitudinally.
8. Tie a long thread on the upper part of the rectus muscle and a short thread on the lower part of rectus abdominis muscle.
9. Transfer the muscle into frog ringer solution containing petridish.
10. Tie the short thread to the hook of the aeration tube and keep the rectus muscle in organ tube.
11. Tie a long thread to a frontal writing lever. The weight on the lever should be 1 gram. The magnification should be between 5 - 7 times.
12. Stabilize the rectus muscle for 30 minutes period.
13. During the stabilization phase replace the frog ringer solution in organ tube at 10 minutes gap.
14. After stabilization for a phase of 30 minutes, switch on the kymograph and record the normal tracing for 30 seconds. At last, 30 seconds period inject 0.1 ml of acetylcholine solution into organ tube and record the tracing for 90 seconds. After 90 seconds turn off kymograph and give 3 - 4 washings of rectus muscle with frog ringer solution.
15. Inject 0.1 ml of solution of acetylcholine in organ tube once again and record the response for 90 seconds.
16. If two equipotent responses are observed with similar doses of acetylcholine, then record the responses with increasing doses of acetylcholine (0.2, 0.4, 0.8 and 1 ml) as shown in Fig. 5.1.

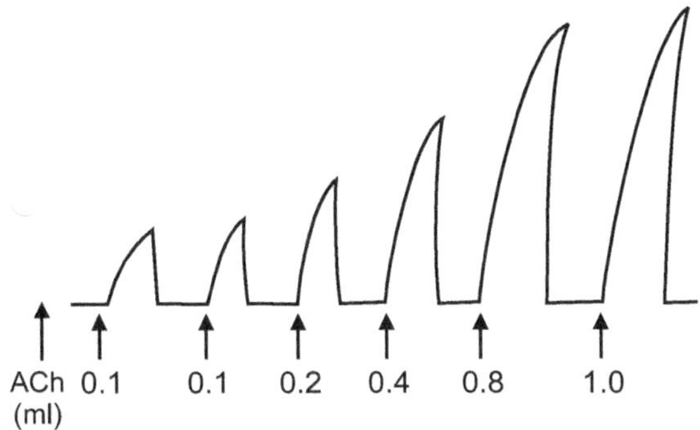

Fig. 5.1: DRC of acetylcholine

17. After fixing the graph measure the height of contraction of the response produced by each dose of acetylcholine and find out the dose which produces maximal response.

Table 5.1: DRC of Acetylcholine on isolated frog rectus abdominis muscle

Sr. No.	Dose of Acetylcholine (ml)	Log dose (Acetylcholine)	Height of contraction (Response) in mm	% Response
1	0.1			
2	0.1			
3	0.2			
4	0.4			
5	0.8			
6	1			

18. Plot a graph showing dose of acetylcholine (ACh) on X-axis and response on Y-axis.

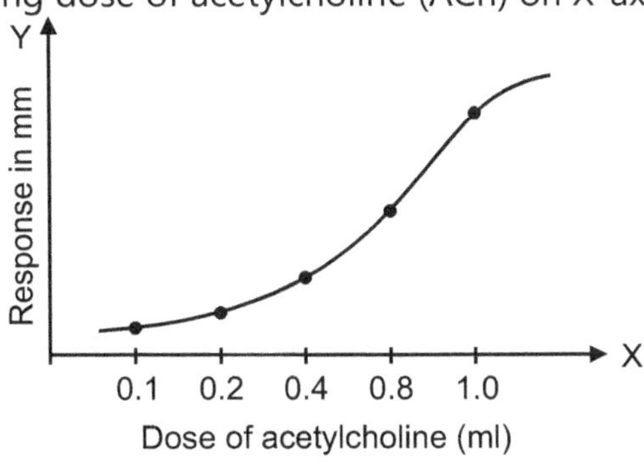

Fig. 5.2

19. Plot the DRC on semilog graph paper taking log dose of agonist on X-axis and % response on Y-axis.

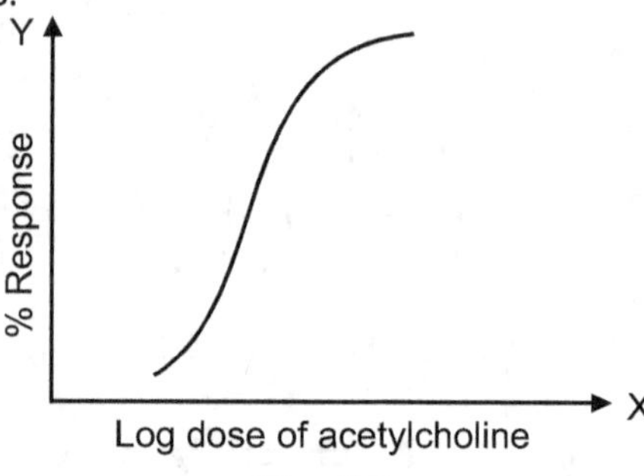

Fig. 5.3

VIVA VOCE QUESTIONS

1. Give the principle in DRC of acetylcholine using frog rectus abdominis muscle.

Ans. Frog rectus abdominis muscle is a voluntary muscle. At the neuromuscular junction, a nerve impulse liberates acetylcholine from the nerve ending into the cleft between nerve fiber as well as muscle. This acetylcholine causes a depolarization of the muscle fiber which in turn sets off a muscle action potential, and contraction of the muscle fiber. The muscle fibers of lower species like frog are multiple innervated and hence nerve stimulation causes persistent depolarization and a prolonged slow contraction of muscle. Local administration of acetylcholine also produces similar effect. Frog rectus abdominis muscle contains nicotinic (N_2) receptors. Acetylcholine works as an agonist.

2. What does dose response curve indicate ?

Ans. Dose response curve indicates

1. Relative potency of the medicine or agonist. The drug is more potent when the curve is more towards the left and the vice versa.

2. Error and reliability (accuracy) of the bioassay is indicated by slope of the curve. Steeper the slope, precise is the assay and vice versa.

3. Explain cumulative DRC.

Ans. The cumulative DRC obtained by increasing the concentration of the drug within the organ tub step by step while not laundry the preceding doses. This method is easy and fewer time overwhelming. It's usually used in those preparations wherever the tissue is slowly getting and slowly restful, but this technique is not fitted to the medication that show fade development. When the doses square measure enlarged in patterned advance (logarithmic intervals) and therefore the response is a plotted against logarithms of doses, the link is termed dose response curve.

4. What are the advantages of logarithmic transformation of doses?

Ans. 1. The linear portion of the sigmoid curve becomes straighter.

2. Comparison of two DRCs is much simpler.

3. Large dose range can be plotted which is otherwise difficult in DRC.

4. The error is distributed all through the graph, free of the dose.

5. What is the time needed for stabilization of tissue?

Ans. 30 minutes are needed for stabilization of tissues.

MULTIPLE CHOICE QUESTIONS (MCQ'S)

1. Select the PSS used in this experiment :

(a) Tyrode solution

(b) Frog ringer solution

(c) De Jalon solution

(d) Krebs solution

2. Select the correct dose of acetylcholine :

(a) 1 mg/ml

(b) 2 mg/ml

(c) 3 mg/ml

(d) 4 mg/ml

3. Which part of frog has been utilized for study?

(a) Ileum

(b) Deuodenum

(c) Jejunum

(d) Rectus abdominis muscle

4. Tension on the frog rectus abdominis muscle is :

(a) 500 mg

(b) 1 gm

(c) 1.5 gm

(d) None of these

5. DRC means :

(a) Drug response curve

(b) Dose response curve

(c) Drug relative curve

(d) Dose relative curve

Answers:

1. (b)	2. (a)	3. (d)	4. (b)	5. (b)

***

Experiment No. 6

Aim: To study effect of physostigmine and atropine on DRC of acetylcholine using frog rectus abdominis muscle and rat ileum respectively.

(A) Effect of Physostigmine (Eserine) on Dose Response Curve of Acetylcholine using frog rectus abdominis muscle:

PRINCIPLE:

Physostigmine is an anticholinesterase substance and it inhibits the metabolic lysis of acetylcholine by preventing the enzyme cholinesterase. Thus when physostigmine is present, more acetylcholine is available for response and the length of contraction of acetylcholine is increased. Due to that action of acetylcholine is potentiated. The DRC of ACh will move towards left because of presence of physostigmine.

REQUIREMENTS:

Equipments and Apparatus: Rotating drum, student organ bath, aerator, frontal writing lever, haemostatic forceps, mariotte bottle, tuberculine syringe, etc.

Animal: Frog

Tissue: Rectus abdominis muscle

Drugs: Acetylcholine (Stock solution - 1 mg/ml)

Physostigmine (Stock solution - 1 mg/ml)

PSS: Frog ringer solution.

Tension on the tissue: 1 gm.

Magnification: 5-7 times

PROCEDURE:

1. Sacrify the frog by pithing or stunning and lay it on its back on the frog dissecting board. Pin the fore limbs.
2. Remove the skin on the abdomen and expose the rectus abdominis muscle.
3. Cut and prepare two rectus muscle preparations from each frog. Tie a thread to upper part and bottom of muscle before separating the muscle from the body of the frog.
4. Place the muscle preparation in vertical arrangement in organ tube which contains frog ringer solution under a tension of 1 gm. It is not required to maintain the bath temperature since it is an amphibian tissue preparation. Bubble the organ tube by using air.
5. Relax the tissue for 45 minutes, during which period wash the tissue with crisp quantum of ringer at any rate multiple times.
6. Record concentration of acetylcholine using either simple sideway or frontal writing lever. 90 second contact time and a total five minutes time cycle is used for proper recording of the responses.
7. Record the CRC of acetylcholine using 4 doses at least.

8.   Add physostigmine (0.2 ml) to the store containing frog ringer and flood the tissue with physostigmine ringer for 30 minutes.

9.   Repeat the concentration response curve of acetylcholine in the presence of physostigmine.

10.   Label and fix both the CRCs.

11.   Plot both the CRCs of acetylcholine (ACh) i.e. in absence and presence of physostigmine.

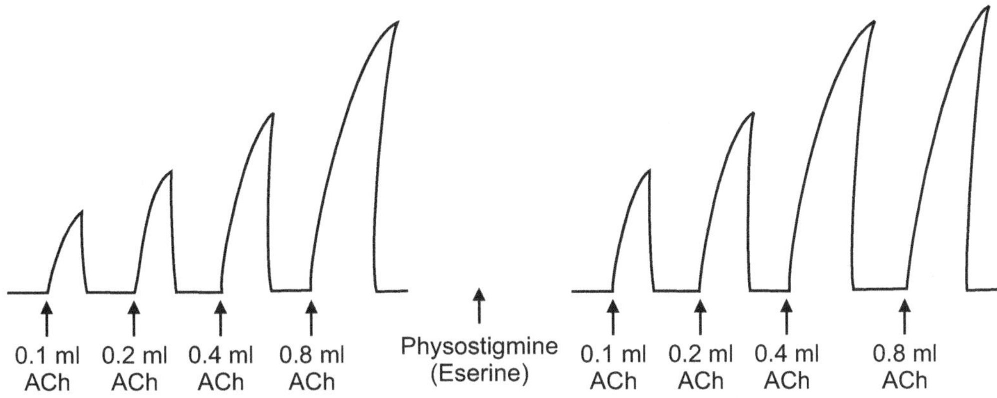

Fig. 6.1: Potentiation of acetylcholine responses by physostigmine (Eserine)

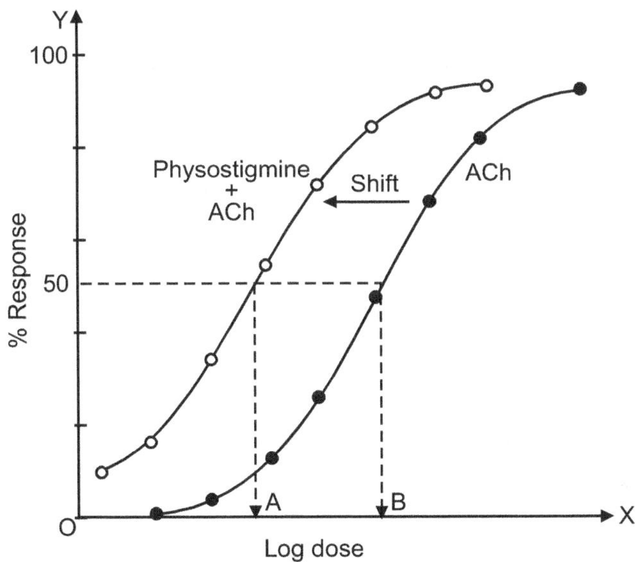

Fig. 6.2: DRC of acetylcholine shifted towards left in presence of physostigmine

12.   Dose proportion (EC50) is determined by looking at the dosages of acetylcholine that is required to create 50% reaction in the nearness and non-appearance of Physostigmine.

13. Note the potentiation the response of acetylcholine and calculate the relative EC50 values.

$$\text{Dose ratio} = \frac{\text{EC50 in presence of Physostigmine}}{\text{EC50 in absence of Physostigmine}}$$

Table 6.1: Dose response relationship of Acetylcholine in absence and presence of Physostigmine

Sr. No.	Dose of ACh	Response of ACh (mm)	Response of ACh in presence of Physostigmine	Log dose	% response of ACh	% Response of ACh in presence of Physostigmine
1.						
2.						
3.						
4.						

(B) Effect of atropine on Dose Response Curve of Acetylcholine using rat ileum:

PRINCIPLE:

Rat ileum is an intestinal smooth muscle. Acetylcholine causes the contraction of smooth muscle by acting on muscarinic receptors. Atropine blocks muscarinic receptors in the smooth muscle. Therefore, atropine blocks acetylcholine induced contractions in ileum of the rat. The CRC of ACh will be moved to the right in the presence of atropine. The nature of antagonism is of competitive type and thus surmountable.

The spontaneous contraction of the preparations is decreased by reducing the calcium content in the physiological solution and maintaining the bath at RT ($23 \pm 2°C$). The muscle preparation obtained from an unstarved rat gives more stable contractions.

REQUIREMENTS:

Equipments and Apparatus: Rotating drum, student organ bath, aerator, frontal writing lever, haemostatic forceps, mariotte bottle, tuberculine syringe, etc.

Animal: Rat (150-200 gm).

Tissue: Ileum.

Drugs: Acetylcholine (Stock solution – 1 mg/ml),

      Atropine (Stock solution - 1 mg/ml)

PSS: Modified ringer (contains less calcium)

Tension on the tissue: 500 mg.

Magnification: 10 times.

PROCEDURE:

1. Sacrify the animal by cervical dislocation.
2. Cut open the abdomen and identify the ileum and place in petridish containing modified ringer's solution.

3. Tenderly wash the lumen and mount the 3 cm long tissue in the organ shower containing adjusted ringer arrangement (pH 7.4) kept up at 25°C and rose with air. The readiness is permitted to equilibrate for 45 minutes under 500 mg pressure.

4. Record the CRC of ACh with the help of frontal writing lever. Contact time of 60 seconds and five minutes time series is kept for proper recording of the responses.

5. Add atropine to modified ringer's solution and irrigate the tissue by atropinised modified ringer for 20 minutes in the reservoir.

6. Repeat the CRC of ACh in presence of atropine.

7. Label and fix the tracing, plot the graph.

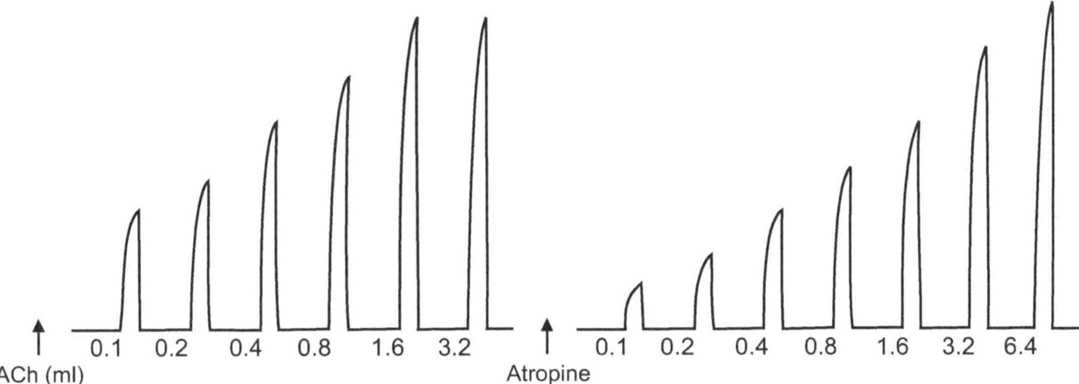

Fig. 6.3: Effect of atropine on DRC of acetylcholine

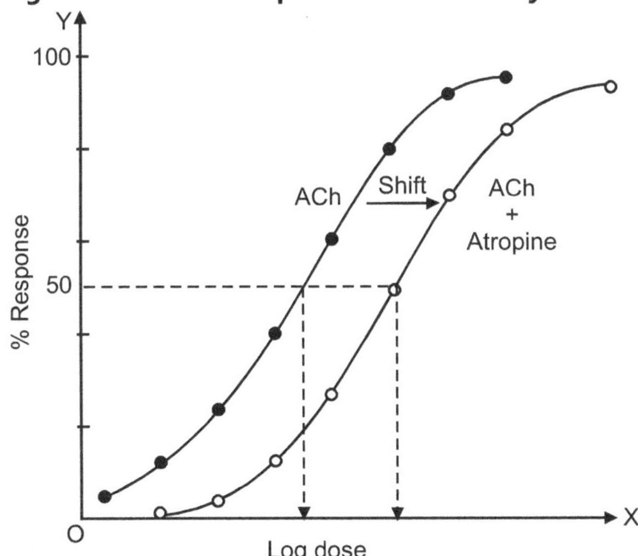

Fig. 6.4: DRC of acetylcholine is shifted towards right in presence of atropine

- **Inference:** Since the focus reaction bend of acetylcholine is moved directly in a parallel manner without concealment of the maximal reaction by atropine, the nature of hostility is aggressive sort.

Table 6.2: Dose response relationship of Acetylcholine in absence and presence of Atropine

Sr. No.	Dose of ACh	Response of ACh (mm)	Response of ACh in presence of Atropine	Log dose	% response of ACh	% Response of ACh in presence of Atropine
1.						
2.						
3.						
4.						

VIVA VOCE QUESTIONS

1. Explain the action of physostigmine on Dose Response Curve of acetylcholine.

Ans. Physostigmine is an anticholinesterase substance and it inhibits the metabolic breakdown of acetylcholine. Therefore the activity of acetylcholine is potentiated. The portion reaction bend of acetylcholine will be moved to one side within the sight of Physostigmine.

2. Explain the action of atropine on Dose Response Curve of acetylcholine.

Ans. Acetylcholine causes the contraction of smooth muscle by acting on muscarinic receptors. Atropine squares muscarinic receptors in the smooth muscle. In this manner, atropine squares acetylcholine actuated withdrawals in rodent ileum. The fixation reaction bend of acetylcholine will be moved to one side within the sight of atropine.

3. Explain the principle in effect of atropine on DRC of acetylcholine using rat ileum.

Ans. Rat ileum is an intestinal smooth muscle. Acetylcholine causes the contraction of smooth muscle by acting on muscarinic receptors. Atropine blocks muscarinic receptors in the smooth muscle. Therefore, atropine blocks acetylcholine induced contractions in ileum of the rat. The CRC of ACh will be moved to the right in the presence of atropine. The nature of antagonism is of competitive type and thus surmountable.

4. Explain the principle in effect of physostigmine on DRC of acetylcholine using frog rectus abdominis muscle.

Ans. Physostigmine is an anticholinesterase substance and it inhibits the metabolic lysis of acetylcholine by preventing the enzyme cholinesterase. Thus when physostigmine is present, more acetylcholine is available for response and the length of contraction of acetylcholine is increased. Due to that, action of acetylcholine is potentiated. The DRC of ACh will move towards left because of presence of physostigmine.

5. Why calcium content is reduced in the PSS?

Ans. For decrease in the spontaneous contractions of preparations/tissue.

MULTIPLE CHOICE QUESTIONS (MCQ'S)

1. Select the correct dose of Physostigmine.

(a) 1 mg/ml	(b) 2 mg/ml
(c) 3 mg/ml	(d) 4 mg/ml

2. Select the correct dose of Atropine.

(a) 0.5 mg/ml	(b) 1 mg/ml
(c) 2 mg/ml	(d) 3 mg/ml

3. Which part of rat is used for experimentation?

(a) Jejunum	(b) Stomach
(c) Ileum	(d) Liver

4. Modified ringer solution contains :

(a) more potassium	(b) less potassium
(c) more calcium	(d) less calcium

5. The DRC of ACh will be moved to the left in the presence of Physostigmine.

(a) True	(b) False

Answers:

1. (a)	2. (b)	3. (c)	4. (d)	5. (a)

***

Experiment No. 7

Aim: Bioassay of histamine using guinea pig ileum by matching method.

INTRODUCTION:

BIOASSAY:

A bioassay is a technique to decide fixation or intensity of a substance by its impact on living cells or tissues. Bioassays were utilized to assess the strength of operators by watching their consequences for living creatures (*in vivo*) or tissues (*in vitro*).

Estimation of the power of a functioning rule in a unit amount of arrangement or discovery and estimation of convergence of a substance in a planning utilizing organic technique is known as natural test or bioassay.

Importance of Bioassay:

Bioassay when contrasted with different strategies for examine like synthetic or physical, are less precise, less detailed, progressively relentless, increasingly problematic and increasingly costly. Anyway bioassay is the main strategy for measure if active principle of drug is unknown or cannot be isolated e.g., insulin, posterior pituitary extract etc.

1. Chemical strategy is either not accessible or if accessible, it is excessively intricate and obtuse or requires higher portion e.g., insulin acetylcholine.
2. Chemical arrangement is not known.
3. Chemical arrangement of medication varies, however, same pharmacological activity and the other way around have.

Matching Bioassay:

It is the least complex sort of bioassay. In this strategy a steady portion of the test is sectioned by fluctuating dosages of standard till the accurate match is acquired between test portion and the standard portion.

At first two reactions of standard are taken. The dosages are balanced to such an extent that one is giving reaction around 20% and other 70% of the most extreme. The reaction of obscure which lies between two reactions of standard portion is taken. The board is rehashed by expanding or diminishing the dosages of standard till three equivalent reactions are gotten. The portion of test is kept steady.

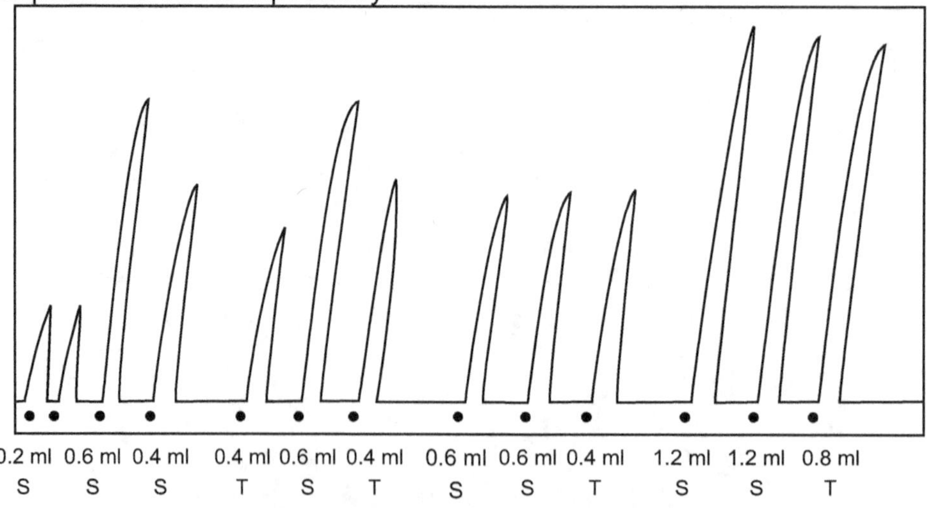

Fig. 7.1: Bioassay of Histamine by matching method

Towards the end, a reaction of the two-fold portion of standard and tests which match each other are taken. These should give equivalent reactions. Grouping of the test can be resolved as pursues:

$$\text{Concentration of unknown} = \frac{\text{Dose of the standard}}{\text{Dose of the test}} \times \text{Concentration of standard}$$

This examine is utilized when the example size is little. Since the test portion not included the chronicle of fixation reaction bend, the affectability of the planning is not thought about. Accordingly, the exactness and dependability are not generally excellent by this technique.

Limitations:

This strategy has following impediments:

1. It involves bigger zone of drum the extent that tracings are concerned.
2. The match is simply emotional, so odds of mistake are there one can't decide them.
3. It does not give any thought regarding portion-reaction relationship.

Advantage:

Matching technique is especially helpful when test size is little and the affectability of the readiness is not steady.

> **Histamine:**

Histamine is a natural nitrogenous compound associated with nearby resistant reactions, just as controlling physiological capacity in the gut and going about as a synapse for the cerebrum, spinal string, and uterus. Histamine is associated with the incendiary reaction and has a focal job as a middle person of tingling. As a component of a resistant reaction to outside pathogens, histamine is created by basophils and by pole cells found in adjacent connective tissues.

REQUIREMENTS:

Equipments and Apparatus: Mariotte bottle, haemostatic forceps, isolated organ bath, aeration tube, isotonic frontal writing lever and recording drum etc.

Animal: Guinea pig.

Tissue: Ileum.

Drug: Histamine (10 µg/ml or 100 µg/ml).

PSS: Tyrode solution.

Tension on the tissue: 1 g.

Magnification: 10 times.

PROCEDURE:

1. Set up the assembly and arrangements are made for experimental condition mentioned above.

2. Sacrify a guinea pig which is fasted overnight by the blow on head and carotid bleeding. Part of ileum is isolated from abdominal cavity after opening.

3. Keep it in petridish which contains tyrode solution. Keep the temperature at 37°C.

4. Separate out the ileum mesentery and clean lumen of ileum by passing warm Tyrode solution through it from pipette held at an angle of about 20-30°.

5. Mount the tissue in mammalian organ bath and associated with isotonic frontal writing lever.

6. Stabilize the tissue for 30 minutes.

7. During the adjustment time frame supplant the tyrode arrangement in the inward organ bath at an interim of 10 minutes.

8. After stabilization (after 30 minutes), switch on the kymograph and record the normal tracing for 30 seconds. At the end of 30 seconds period, inject 0.1 ml of histamine solution into the inner organ tube and record the tracing for 90 seconds. At the end of 90 seconds turn off the kymograph and give 3-4 washings of ileum with tyrode solution.

9. Initially record 2 responses of standard. Adjust the doses such that one is giving response approximately 20% and other 70% of the maximum. Take the response of unknown which lies between two responses of standard dose.

10. Repeat the process by increasing or decreasing the doses of standard till three equal responses are obtained. Keep the dose of test sample constant.

11. Finally, take a response of the double dose of standard and test which match each other. These should give equal responses.

12. Determine the concentration of the test sample as follows:

$$\text{Concentration of unknown} = \frac{\text{Dose of the standard}}{\text{Dose of the test}} \times \text{Concentration of standard}$$

VIVA VOCE QUESTIONS

1. Define Bioassay.

Ans. A bioassay is a technique to decide fixation or intensity of a substance by its impact on living cells or tissues. Bioassays were utilized to assess the strength of operators by watching their consequences on living creatures (in vivo) or tissues (*in vitro*).

Estimation of the power of a functioning rule in a unit amount of arrangement or discovery and estimation of convergence of a substance in a planning utilizing organic technique is known as natural test or bioassay.

2. Give importance of bioassay.

Ans. Bioassay when contrasted with different strategies for examine like synthetic or physical, are less precise, less detailed, progressively relentless, increasingly problematic and increasingly costly. Anyway bioassay is the main strategy for measure if active principle of drug is unknown or cannot be isolated e.g., insulin, posterior pituitary extract etc.

1. Chemical strategy is either not accessible or if accessible, it is excessively intricate and obtuse or requires higher portion e.g., insulin acetylcholine.

2. Chemical arrangement is not known.

3. Chemical arrangement of medication varies, however, same pharmacological activity and the other way around have.

3. Write limitations of matching bioassay.

Ans. This strategy has following impediments:

1. It involves bigger zone of drum the extent that tracings are concerned.

2. The match is simply emotional, so odds of mistake are there one can't decide them.

3. It does not give any thought regarding portion-reaction relationship.

4. Explain matching method.

Ans. It is the least complex sort of bioassay. In this strategy a steady portion of the test is sectioned by fluctuating dosages of standard till the accurate match is acquired between test portion and the standard portion.

At first two reactions of standard are taken. The dosages are balanced to such an extent that one is giving reaction around 20% and other 70% of the most extreme. The reaction of obscure which lies between two reactions of standard portion is taken. The board is rehashed by expanding or diminishing the dosages of standard till three equivalent reactions are gotten. The portion of test is kept steady.

Towards the end, a reaction of the two-fold portion of standard and tests which match each other are taken. These should give equivalent reactions. Grouping of the test can be resolved as pursues:

$$\text{Concentration of unknown} = \frac{\text{Dose of the standard}}{\text{Dose of the test}} \times \text{Concentration of standard}$$

5. Give the significance of matching bioassay.

Ans. Matching method is mainly helpful when the sensitivity of the research is not steady.

MULTIPLE CHOICE QUESTIONS (MCQ'S)

1. Which animal is used for bioassay of histamine?

   (a) Hamster   (b) Rabbit

   (c) Frog   (d) Guinea Pig

2. Select correct tension on the tissue :

   (a) 500 mg   (b) 1 gm

   (c) 1.5 gm   (d) 2 gm

3. **Which PSS is used for histamine bioassay?**
   (a) Tyrode solution (b) Krebs solution
   (c) De Jalon solution (d) Frog ringer solution

4. **Magnification value for bioassay of histamine is**
   (a) 2 times (b) 5 times
   (c) 7 times (d) 10 times

5. **Matching method is particularly useful if the sensitivity of the preparation is stable.**
   (a) True (b) False

Answers:

| 1. (d) | 2. (b) | 3. (a) | 4. (d) | 5. (b) |

***

Experiment No. 8

Aim: Bioassay of oxytocin using rat uterine horn by interpolation method.

INTRODUCTION:

Oxytocin:

Oxytocin is a peptide hormone and neuropeptide. Oxytocin is usually made by the paraventricular nucleus of the hypothalamus and released by the posterior pituitary. It is responsible in social bonding, sexual reproduction, in childbirth process. Oxytocin is secreted in blood circulation, in response to stretching of the cervix and uterus during labor. This helps with birth and production of milk. Oxytocin was revealed by Henry Dale in 1906.

Interpolation Method:

In this type of bioassay, a CRC of standard substance is first established. Then 2-3 responses of test substance are recorded. The selection of the test responses should be such that they lie on the linear portion of the CRC of the standard drug.

PRINCIPLE:

The rat uterine preparations are usually employed for bioassay of oxytocin. The sensitivity of the uterus to oxytocin depends upon the estrus cycles. The various stages of estrus cycle are examined by preparing the vaginal smear and observing under microscope. An adult (2-3 months) female rat has an estrus cycle of 5 days. The estrus cycle can be categorised in four different stages as follows:

1. **Estrus:** It is distinguished by increased running activity, quivering of ears and lordosis in the company of another rat. The vaginal smear shows epithelial cells (cornified) only. It ends within 9-15 hours, with ovulation.

2. **Metaestrus:** It occurs shortly after ovulation. Leucocytes starts appearing in this stage and predominate over cornified epithelial cells. It lasts for about 15-18 hours.

3. **Diestrus:** This stage lasts for 60-70 hours. Vaginal smear shows only leucocytes.

4. **Proestrus:** It is of about 12 hours, distinguished by epithelial cells (nucleated) either singly or in groups.

If the rat is not in estrus, this phase is provoked by the oestrogen preparation administration, stilboestrol (0.1 mg/kg, sc, 24 hours before).

Estrus uterus is highly sensitive to oxytocin and hence prepared for bioassay, however high spontaneous uterus contraction in estrus stage may pose difficulty in carrying out the experiment. Conversely, in diestrus is relatively less sensitive to oxytocin.

Standard Preparation and Unit:

It is the 4th international standard established in 1978. It consists of freeze dried synthetic oxytocin peptide with human albumin and citric acid (supplied in ampoules containing 12.5 units).

REQUIREMENTS:

Equipments and Apparatus: Isotonic frontal writing lever, isolated organ bath, aeration tube, and recording drum Mariotte bottle etc.

Animal: Female rat (120-150 g).

Tissue: Uterine horn.

Drugs: Estradiol (100 µg/kg).

      Oxytocin (0.05 – 0.1 unit).

PSS: De Jalon Solution.

Tension on the tissue: 500 mg.

PROCEDURE:

1. Select the female rat weighing in between 120-150 g and examine the vaginal smear under microscope for confirmation of estrus cycle and stage (day).
2. If the rat is not in estrus then, before 24 hours of experiment administer 100 µg/kg of estradiol by intramuscular route and confirm the estrus stage by examining vaginal smear on the day of experiment.
3. Sacrify the rat; isolate uterine horn and mount in organ tube which contains de Jalon solution. Maintain the organ bath at temperature of 32°C and is oxygenate it.
4. Record the contractions of uterine horn by a frontal writing lever on smoked paper fixed on the slowly revolving drum.
5. Add standard oxytocin dose (0.05-0.1 unit) in inner tube. This causes contraction of uterus and when contraction is complete, drain out the solution present in the bath and run in the new solution and allow the muscle to relax.
6. Record the CRC due to oxytocin using standard oxytocin solution.
7. Record response due to graded dose of the test substance. See that these responses would fall on linear portion of the CRC for standard solution.
8. Label and fix the tracing.
9. Plot the CRC due to standard oxytocin solution. Measure the heights of the contractions (response) due to different doses (A and B) of the test solution. Read the corresponding concentration from standard curve.

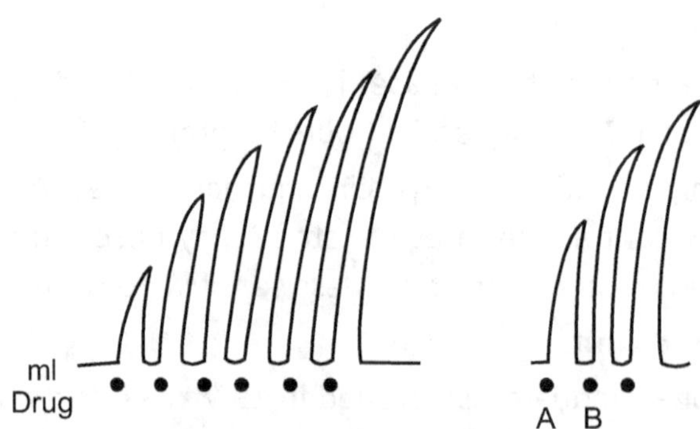

Fig. 8.1: Representative tracing of interpolation bioassay

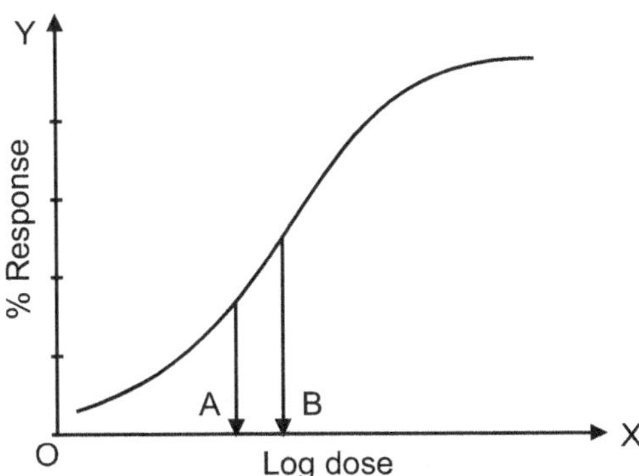

Fig. 8.2: Estimation of concentration of test sample by interpolation bioassay

VIVA VOCE QUESTIONS

1. Explain oxytocin.

Ans. Oxytocin is a peptide hormone and neuropeptide. Oxytocin is usually made by the paraventricular nucleus of the hypothalamus and released by the posterior pituitary. It is responsible in social bonding, sexual reproduction, in childbirth process. Oxytocin is secreted in blood circulation, in response to stretching of the cervix and uterus during labour. This helps with birth and production of milk. Oxytocin was revealed by Henry Dale in 1906.

2. Explain Interpolation method.

Ans. In this type of bioassay a CRC of standard substance is first established. Then 2-3 responses of test substance are recorded. The selection of the test responses should be such that they lie on the linear portion of the CRC of the standard drug.

3. Give the principle in bioassay of oxytocin.

Ans. The rat uterine preparations are usually employed for bioassay of oxytocin. The sensitivity of the uterus to oxytocin depends upon the estrus cycles. The various stages of estrus cycle are examined by preparing the vaginal smear and observing under microscope. An adult (2-3 months) female rat has an estrus cycle of 5 days.

4. Write the phases of estrus cycle.

Ans. The estrus cycle can be categorized in four different phases as follows:

1. **Estrus:** It is distinguished by increased running activity, quivering of ears and lordosis in the company of another rat. The vaginal smear shows epithelial cells (cornified) only. It ends within 9-15 hours, with ovulation.

2. **Metaestrus:** It occurs shortly after ovulation. Leucocytes starts appearing in this stage and predominate over cornified epithelial cells. It lasts for about 15-18 hours.

3. **Diestrus:** This stage lasts for 60-70 hours. Vaginal smear shows only leucocytes.

4. **Proestrus:** It is of about 12 hours, distinguished by epithelial cells (nucleated) either singly or in groups.

5. **Who discovered oxytocin?**

Ans. Oxytocin was discovered by Henry Dale in 1906.

MULTIPLE CHOICE QUESTIONS (MCQ'S)

1. **Which animal is used for this experiment?**
   - (a) Rabbit
   - (b) Rat
   - (c) Frog
   - (d) Guinea Pig

2. **Which PSS is used for this experiment?**
   - (a) Frog ringer solution
   - (b) Krebs solution
   - (c) Tyrode solution
   - (d) De Jalon solution

3. **Select the dose (standard) of oxytocin.**
   - (a) 0.05 - 0.1 unit
   - (b) 0.05 - 0.2 unit
   - (c) 0.05 - 0.3 unit
   - (d) 0.05 - 0.4 unit

4. **Which tissue of the animal is used for this experiment?**
   - (a) Duodenum
   - (b) Uterine horn
   - (c) Ileum
   - (d) Fundus strip

5. **If the rat is not in estrus, it can be induced by the administration of oestrogen preparation.**
   - (a) True
   - (b) False

Answers:

1. (b)	2. (d)	3. (a)	4. (b)	5. (a)

****

9. Select a dose of test sample t_1 which is likely to produce a response less than the response produced by S_2 dose of standard as shown below.

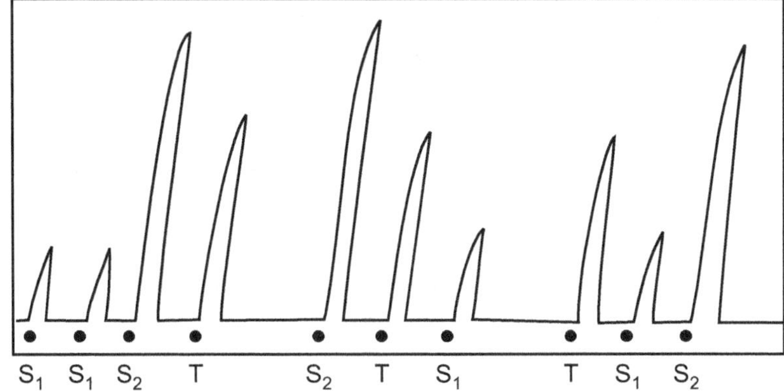

Fig. 9.1: Bioassay of Serotonin by three-point method

10. Measure the height of contraction produced by S_1 dose as S_1.
11. Measure the height of contraction produced by S_2 dose as S_2.
12. Measure the height of contraction produced by t_1 dose as T.
13. Calculate the potency of the test solution:

$$\text{Concentration of unknown} = \frac{n_1}{t} \times \text{Antilog} \left\{ \frac{T - S_1}{S_2 - S_1} \times \log \frac{n_2}{n_1} \right\} C_s$$

Table 9.1: Mean responses of standard and test solution of Serotonin

Sr. No.	Different responses	Height of different responses (mm)			
		1	2	3	Mean
1.	S_1				
2.	S_2				
3.	T				

VIVA VOCE QUESTIONS

1. Explain three-point bioassay.

Ans. In three-point bioassay method, 2 doses of standard and 1 dose of test are used. The DRC of standard and test samples is first taken from responses due to graded doses.

2. Discuss serotonin.

Ans. Serotonin is also known as 5-hydroxytryptamine, or 5-HT. It is essentially found in the brain, guts, and blood platelets. Serotonin is utilized to transmit messages between nerve cells, it is believed to be dynamic in tightening smooth muscles, and it adds to prosperity and satisfaction, in addition to other things. As the antecedent for melatonin, it controls the body's rest wake cycles and the inner clock. It is thought to assume a job in hunger, the feelings, and engine, intellectual, and autonomic capacities.

3. **Write the principle of bioassay of serotonin using rat fundus strip by three point method.**

Ans. Rat fundus is extremely sensitive tissue for examination of several naturally occurring substances like 5 – HT, histamine, acetylcholine and bradykinin. Unlike the intestinal smooth muscle this preparation is slow contracting and slow relaxing type. Rat fundus is usually used for the bioassay of serotonin. The fundus (upper portion of stomach) is grey in colour and therefore, easily identified from pyloric part (pink in colour). A zig zag preparation of the fundus strip is prepared in an attempt to expose maximum part of tissue to drug.

The tissue is sensitive to 1 µg/ml of serotonin, 0.05-1 µg/ml of histamine and 0.2-0.5 µg/ml of acetylcholine, respectively.

4. **Give the formula for three-point bioassay.**

Ans. Concentration of unknown $= \dfrac{n_1}{t} \times \text{Antilog} \left\{ \dfrac{T - S_1}{S_2 - S_1} \times \log \dfrac{n_2}{n_1} \right\} C_s$

5. **Write another name of serotonin.**

Ans. Another name for serotonin is 5-hydroxytryptamine, or 5-HT.

MULTIPLE CHOICE QUESTIONS (MCQ'S)

1. **Which animal is used for bioassay of serotonin?**
   (a) Rat
   (b) Rabbit
   (c) Frog
   (d) Guinea Pig

2. **Which PSS is used for bioassay of serotonin?**
   (a) Frog ringer solution
   (b) Krebs solution
   (c) Tyrode solution
   (d) De Jalon solution

3. **Select the correct concentration of serotonin :**
   (a) 0.1 µg/ml
   (b) 0.2 µg/ml
   (c) 0.5 µg/ml
   (d) 1.0 µg/ml

4. **Which tissue of the animal is used for bioassay of serotonin?**
   (a) Duodenum
   (b) Jejunum
   (c) Ileum
   (d) Rat fundus strip

5. **A zig zag preparation of the fundus strip is prepared so as to expose maximum portion of the tissue to drug.**
   (a) True
   (b) False

Answers:

1. (a)	2. (b)	3. (c)	4. (d)	5. (a)

***

Experiment No. 10

Aim: Bioassay of acetylcholine using rat ileum/colon by four point bioassay.

INTRODUCTION:

➢ **Four Point Bioassay:**

In four-point bioassay two reactions of the standard medication and two reactions of the test substance are taken. The choice of two reactions of the standard ought to be to such an extent that they lie on the straight segment of the fixation reaction bend and furthermore the proportion between the dosages ought to be ideally 1 : 2. The determination of the test reaction is dictated by hit and preliminary strategy with the goal that the reaction falls on the direct piece of the bend. Utilizing the Latin square plan the reactions are recorded in an irregular manner.

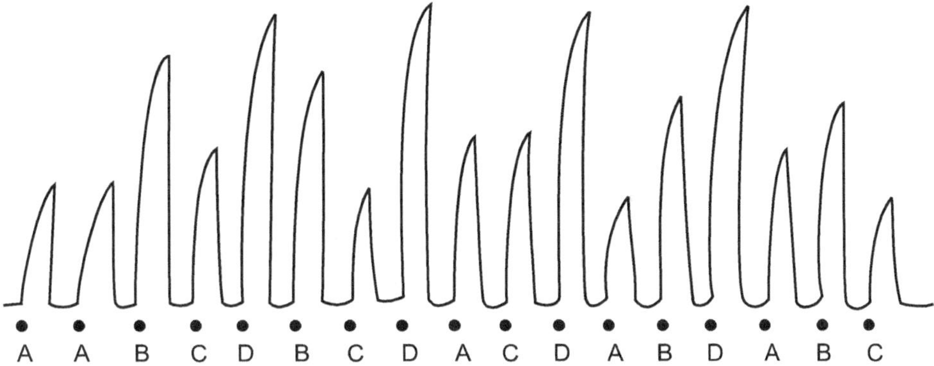

Fig. 10.1: Four-point bioassay

Advantages:

1. The precision, reliability and reproducibility of this assay method are very high.
2. It is generally employed for determination of the concentration of unknown sample.

➢ **Acetylcholine:**

It is the neurotransmitter of parasympathetic, somatic nerves and autonomic ganglia. Acetylcholine has both muscarinic and nicotinic activity. It's actions include:

1. Decrease in heart rate and cardiac output.
2. Decrease in blood pressure.
3. Miscellaneous:
    (i)   In GIT, ACh increases salivary secretion as well as intestinal secretion and motility.
    (ii) It increases bronchial secretions.
    (iii) Acetylcholine is responsible for constriction of pupil (miosis).

REQUIREMENTS:

Equipments and Apparatus: Kymograph, student's organ bath, Frontal writing lever, scissors, forceps, thread, plasticine, pithing needle, etc.

Animal: Rat.

Tissue: Ileum.

Drug: Acetylcholine (Stock solution −100 µg/ml).

Test solution of acetylcholine.

PSS: De Jalon/Krebs solution.

Tension on the tissue: 500 mg.

Magnification: 10 times.

PROCEDURE:

1. Set up the assembly.

2. Sacrify the rat.

3. Abdominal pouch is quickly opened and the ileum is isolated. Transfer it in petridish which contains De Jalon/Krebs solution maintained at 37°C.

4. Take away the mesentery of ileum and clean ileum by passing warm PSS by using pipette (pipette held at angle about 20-30°).

5. Mount the piece of ileum in mammalian organ tube and connect it to isotonic frontal lever. The tissue should be permitted to balance out for 30 minutes.

6. Record the dose dependant response of standard solution of acetylcholine as shown in Fig. 10.2.

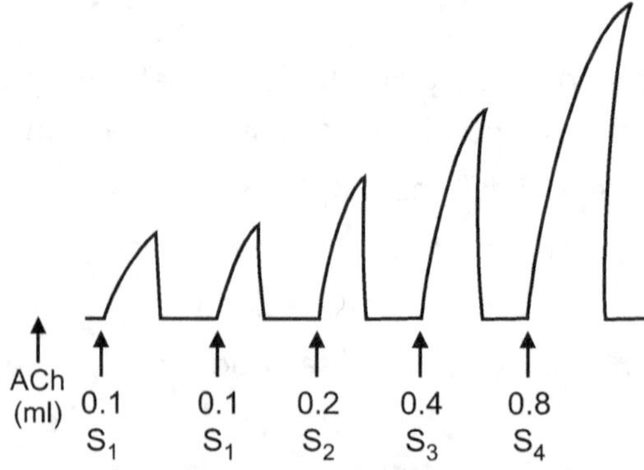

Fig. 10.2: Dose response curve of standard solution of acetylcholine

7. Trace response of the given test dose of acetylcholine as shown in Fig. 10.3.

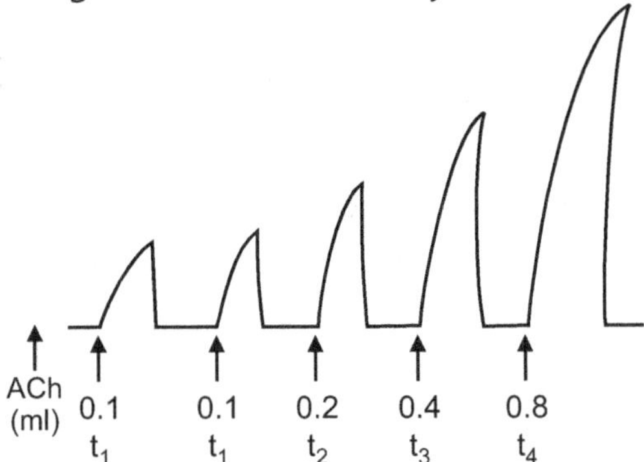

Fig. 10.3: Dose response curve of test solution of acetylcholine

8. Select two standard doses of acetylcholine solution which produce submaximal response (1 : 2 ratio).
9. Select two test doses of acetylcholine solution which produce submaximal response.
10. Administer the S_1, S_2, t_1 and t_2 doses four times in a randomized fashion (Latin square design).

$$S_1 = A, S_2 = B, t_1 = C, t_2 = D$$

1st Sequence	2nd Sequence	3rd Sequence	4th Sequence
ABCD	BCDA	CDAB	DABC

11. Measure the height of concentration produced by S_1 (A) and S_2 (B), doses of acetylcholine and calculate the mean response as S_1 and S_2 respectively.
12. Measure the height of concentration produced by t_1 (C) and t_2 (D) doses of acetylcholine and calculate the mean response as T_1 and T_2 respectively.
13. Plot a graph by taking log dose of ACh standard as well as test on X-axis and response on Y-axis as shown in Fig. 10.4.

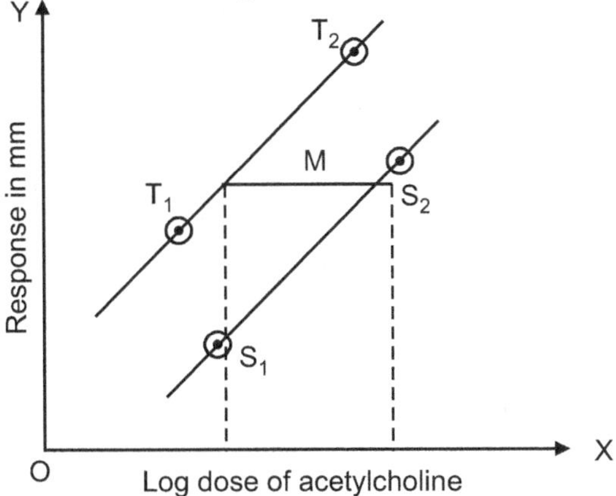

Fig. 10.4

M = Log potency ratio

Antilog of M = Potency ratio

14. Potency ratio can also be calculated by using following formula:

$$\text{Potency of the test} = \frac{n_1}{t_1} \times \text{Antilog} \left\{ \frac{(S_1 + S_2) - (T_1 + T_2)}{(S_2 + T_2) - (S_1 + T_1)} \right\} \times \log \frac{n_2}{n_1}$$

OBSERVATIONS:

Table 10.1: Mean responses of standard and test solution of Acetylcholine

Sr. No.	Different responses	Height of different responses (mm)				
		1	2	3	4	Mean
1.	S_1					
2.	S_2					
3.	T_1					
4.	T_2					

VIVA VOCE QUESTIONS

1. Explain four-point bioassay.

Ans. In four point bioassay two reactions of the standard medication and two reactions of the test substance are taken. The choice of two reactions of the standard ought to be to such an extent that they lie on the straight segment of the fixation reaction bend and furthermore the proportion between the dosages ought to be ideally 1 : 2. The determination of the test reaction is dictated by hit and preliminary strategy with the goal that the reaction falls on the direct piece of the bend. Utilizing the Latin square plan the reactions are recorded in an irregular manner.

2. What are the advantages of four-point bioassay.

Ans. (i) The precision, reliability and reproducibility of this assay method are very high.

(ii) It is generally employed for determination of the concentration of unknown sample.

3. Give the formula for four-point bioassay.

Ans. Potency of the test $= \dfrac{n_1}{t_1} \times \text{Antilog} \left\{ \dfrac{(S_1 + S_2) - (T_1 + T_2)}{(S_2 + T_2) - (S_1 + T_1)} \right\} \times \log \dfrac{n_2}{n_1}$

4. Give the effect of acetylcholine on GIT.

Ans. In GIT, acetylcholine increases salivary secretion as well as intestinal secretion and motility.

5. Write pharmacological actions of acetylcholine.

Ans. (i) Reduces HR and CO.

(ii) Reduces BP.

(iii) Increases bronchial secretions.

(iv) Acetylcholine is responsible for constriction of pupil (miosis) etc.

MULTIPLE CHOICE QUESTIONS (MCQ'S)

1. **Which animal is used for bioassay of acetylcholine?**

   (a) Rat

   (b) Rabbit

   (c) Frog

   (d) Guinea Pig

2. **Which PSS is used for bioassay of acetylcholine?**

   (a) Krebs solution

   (b) Frog ringer solution

   (c) Tyrode solution

   (d) De Jalon solution

3. **Select the correct concentration of acetylcholine :**

   (a) 50 µg/ml

   (b) 100 µg/ml

   (c) 150 µg/ml

   (d) 200 µg/ml

4. **The tissue is permitted to balance out for 30 minutes.**

   (a) True

   (b) False

5. **In four-point bioassay method, precision, reliability and reproducibility are very low.**

   (a) True

   (b) False

Answers:

1. (a)	2. (c)	3. (b)	4. (a)	5. (b)

***

Experiment No. 11

Aim: Determination of pA_2 value of prazosin using rat anococcygeus muscle (by Schilds plot method).

INTRODUCTION:

➢ **pA_2 value:**

The pA_x value is calculated as the negative logarithm of the molar concentration of the antagonist required to reduce the effect of multiple dose (x) of the agonist to that of single dose in the absence of antagonism. The use of pA_x value is convenient method for evaluating competitive antagonism. Higher the pA_x value, more potent is the antagonist.

pA_x value according to the Schilds is defined as negative logarithm to base 10 of the molar concentration of an antagonist which reduces the effect of a multiple dose of an active drug to that of single dose. The determination of pA_2 (x = 2) and pA_{10} (x = 10) values has wider applications. If the difference between these two values is found to be 0.95 or very near (0.8-1.2), the antagonism is likely to be of competitive type. An antagonist acting on the same receptor will have the same pA_2 value in all tissue or organ preparations.

➢ **pA_2 Analysis and Schilds Plot:**

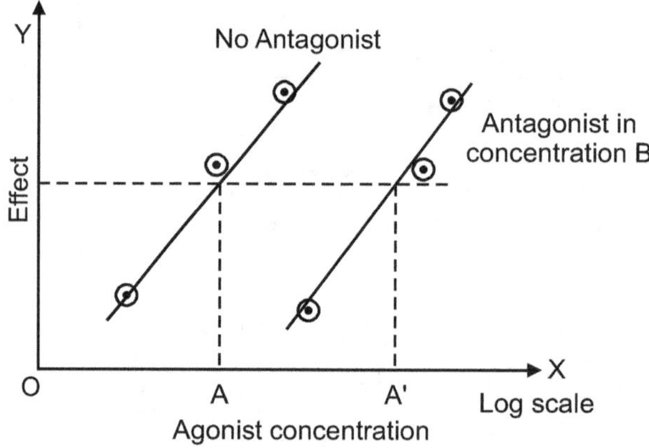

Fig. 11.1: Agonist dose response curve

H. O. Schild proposed a scale i.e. pA scale to determine drug antagonism in 1947. The pA_2 is a measure of the affinity of a competitive antagonist for its receptor. The determination of the pA_2 is made from experiments in which a fixed concentration of the antagonist is used along with graded concentrations of an agonist acting on the same receptor. The presence of the antagonist shifts the agonist dose-response curve to the right.

➢ **Rat Anococcygeus Muscle:**

Rat anococcygeus muscle is smooth muscle which is attached to the bone. This muscle arises independently from one or more, usually two upper coccygeal vertebrae in the middle of pelvic cavity. The muscles at their origin lie near to one another and at the back of the terminal colon. They then pass caudally and ventrally lying first behind and sweep around the lateral part of the colon, about 0.5-1 cm short of anal margin. The muscles can be easily and quickly dissected out and are about 3 cm long, 150-300 μm thick and about 0.5 cm broad. The muscles in male rat are noticeably stronger, heavier and broader than those in females, and form a pronounced ventral bar in front of the colon, a feature hardly developed in females.

Rat anococcygeus muscle has a thick adrenergic innervations conveyed all through the muscle yet evidently no cholinergic innervations.

The muscle contracts to noradrenaline, acetylcholine, 5 – HT, yet not to histamine.

➢ **Prazosin:**

Prazosin is a sympatholytic medication used to treat the hypertension, anxiety, and posttraumatic stress disorder (PTSD). Prazosin is a α_1-blocker that acts as an inverse agonist at α_1 adrenergic receptors. These receptors are found on vascular smooth muscle, where they are responsible for the vasoconstrictive action of norepinephrine. They are also found throughout the central nervous system.

➢ **Norepinephrine:**

It is also called noradrenaline (NA). It is an organic chemical in the catecholamine family that functions in the brain and body as a hormone and neurotransmitter.

REQUIREMENTS:

Equipments and Apparatus: Student organ bath, aerator, frontal writing lever, lever holder, haemostatic forceps, mariotte bottle, rubber tubes, tuberculine syringe, pithing needle, scissor and forceps etc.

Animal: Rat.

Tissue: Anococcygeus muscle.

Drugs: Prazosin (1 μg/ml, Mol. wt. – 383.401) and Norepinephrine (10 μg/ml, Mol. wt. – 169.18).

PSS: Krebs solution.

Tension: 1 gm.

Magnification: 10 times.

PROCEDURE:

1. Set the assembly and make the arrangements for experimental condition.
2. Keep the rat for overnight fasting and scarify it as per CPCSEA guidelines. Quickly open the abdominal cavity and isolate anococcygeus muscle. Transfer the isolated muscle in petridish which contains Krebs solution (maintained at 37°C).
3. Mount the tissue in mammalian organ bath and connect to isolated frontal writing lever.
4. Stabilize the tissue for 30 minutes, in between that give the repeated washes after every 10 minutes.
5. Take the DRC of norepinephrine using graded dose till the maximum response is obtained.

6. Identify 2 doses bearing 1 : 2 dose ratio producing submaximal response (A, 2A) for pA_2 determination.

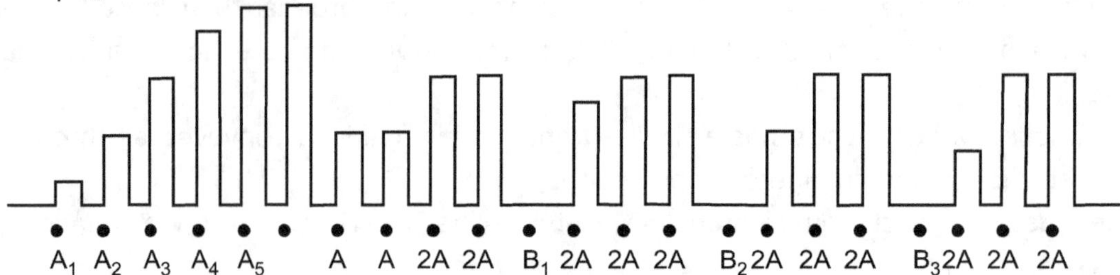

Fig. 11.2: Principle of pA_2 determination

7. Standardize the tissue by selecting the doses of norepinephrine. A tissue is said to be standardize when it responds same to the dose of an agonist after repetition.

8. Record the concentrations of double dose of norepinephrine (2A) in the presence of different concentrations (B_1, B_2, B_3) of prazosin.

9. Consider the response due to the double dose of norepinephrine (2A) i.e., before adding the prazosin as 100 % response. Determine the corresponding % response to this dose of norepinephrine (2A) in the presence of different concentrations of prazosin.

10. Plot a graph representing negative log of molar concentration of prazosin employed along X-axis and % response along Y-axis.

    pA_2 value is defined as the negative log of molar concentration of prazosin required to reduce the effect of a dose 2A to A, respectively.

11. Read out pA_2 value for prazosin from the graph directly. It corresponds to the % response obtained with the half dose of prazosin (A).

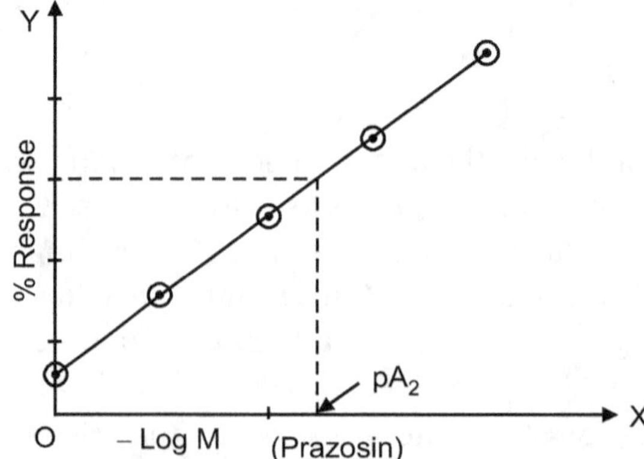

Fig. 11.3: Estimation of pA_2 value for prazosin

Table 11.1: pA_2 value of prazosin using noradrenaline as agonist

Sr. No.	Molar concentration of Noradrenaline	Molar concentration of Prazosin	Response (mm)	Log	% Response
1.	A				
2.	2A				
3.	2A	B_1			
3.	2A	B_2			
4.	2A	B_3			

Where, A and 2A are two doses of noradrenaline obtained from linear range of DRC.

B_1, B_2, B_3 are the increased concentrations of prazosin.

VIVA VOCE QUESTIONS

1. Explain pA_2 value.

Ans. pA_2 value is defined as the negative log of molar concentration of drug required to reduce the effect of a dose 2A to A, respectively.

The pA_x value is calculated as the negative logarithm of the molar concentration of the antagonist required to reduce the effect of multiple dose (x) of the agonist to that of single dose in the absence of antagonist. The use of pA_x value is convenient method for evaluating competitive antagonism. Higher the pA_x value, more potent is the antagonist.

pA_x value according to the Schilds is defined as negative logarithm to base 10 of the molar concentration of an antagonist which reduces the effect of a multiple dose of an active drug to that of single dose. The determination of pA_2 (x = 2) and pA_{10} (x = 10) values has wider applications. If the difference between these two values is found to be 0.95 or very near (0.8-1.2), the antagonism is likely to be of competitive type. An antagonist acting on the same receptor will have the same pA_2 value in all tissue or organ preparations.

2. Explain rat anococcygeus muscle.

Ans. Rat anococcygeus muscle is smooth muscle which is attached to the bone. This muscle arises independently from one or more, usually two upper coccygeal vertebrae in the middle of pelvic cavity. The muscles at their origin lie near to one another and at the back of the terminal colon. They then pass caudally and ventrally lying first behind and sweep around the lateral part of the colon, about 0.5 – 1 cm short of anal margin. The muscles can be easily and quickly dissected out and are about 3 cm long, 150 - 300 µm thick and about 0.5 cm broad. The muscles in male rat are noticeably stronger, heavier and broader than those in females, and form a pronounced ventral bar in front of the colon, a feature hardly developed in females.

3. Explain norepinephrine.

Ans. It is also called noradrenaline (NA). It is an organic chemical in the catecholamine family that functions in the brain and body as a hormone and neurotransmitter.

4. Give MOA of prazosin.

Ans. Prazosin is a α_1-blocker that acts as an inverse agonist at α_1-adrenergic receptors.

5. Write uses of prazosin.

Ans. Prazosin is a sympatholytic medication, used to treat the hypertension, anxiety, and posttraumatic stress disorder (PTSD), etc.

MULTIPLE CHOICE QUESTIONS (MCQ'S)

1. **Which animal is used to determine pA_2 value of prazosin?**
   - (a) Rat
   - (b) Rabbit
   - (c) Frog
   - (d) Guinea Pig

2. **Which tissue of animal is used for determination of pA_2 value of prazosin?**
   - (a) Duodenum
   - (b) Jejunum
   - (c) Ileum
   - (d) Anococcygeus muscles

3. **Select the PSS used to determine pA_2 value of prazosin :**
   - (a) De Jalon solution
   - (b) Krebs solution
   - (c) Tyrode solution
   - (d) Frog ringer solution

4. **Effect of NE is :**
   - (a) It increases heart rate.
   - (b) It increases blood pressure.
   - (c) It increases arousal and alertness.
   - (d) All of these.

5. **If the variation between pA_2 and pA_{10} is 0.95 or very near (0.8-1.2), the antagonism is likely to be of competitive type.**
   - (a) True
   - (b) False

Answers:

1. (a)	2. (d)	3. (b)	4. (d)	5. (a)

★★★

Experiment No. 12

Aim: Determination of pD_2 value using guinea pig ileum.

PRINCIPLE:

The EC50 value describes relative potency of the drugs. Lower the EC50 value, more potent is the drug. Sometimes the same is indicated as pD_2 value which is defined as negative log of molar concentration of the drug producing 50% of maximal response. If pD_2 value is high, then the potency is also high. In calculating the pD_2 value, the % of the maximum response produced by each dose (concentration) is plotted against log molar concentration of the drug and the concentration producing 50% response is read as pD_2 value. The EC50 or pD_2 values are used to express the affinity of a drug. Both the values can be interconvertible employing a simple equation i.e. if EC50 is expressed as $(m \times 10^{-n})$, then $pD_2 = n - \log m$.

Dose ratio (EC50) is calculated by comparing the doses of ACh, needed to produce 50% response in presence and absence of drug.

REQUIREMENTS:

Equipments and Apparatus: Student organ bath, aerator, frontal writing lever, mariotte bottle, rubber tubes, tuberculine syringe, pithing needle, scissor, forceps etc.

Animal: Guinea pig.

Tissue: Ileum.

PSS: Tyrode solution.

Drug: Acetylcholine (Stock solution –1 mg/ml).

Tension on the tissue: 500 mg.

Magnification: 10 times.

PROCEDURE:

1. Set up the assembly and make the arrangements for experimental condition mentioned above.
2. Sacrify a guinea pig which is fasted overnight as per CPCSEA guidelines. Quickly open the abdominal pouch and isolate the ileum.
3. Transfer it in petridish which contains Tyrode solution (maintained at 37°C).
4. Remove the mesentery of ileum and clean the lumen of ileum by passing warm Tyrode solution through it from pipette held at an angle of about 20-30°.
5. Mount the tissue in mammalian organ tube which is attached to isotonic frontal writing lever.
6. Stabilize ileum for 30 minutes.
7. During the stabilization period replace the tyrode solution in the inner tube bath at gap of 10 minutes.
8. After 30 minutes stabilization, switch on the kymograph and record the normal tracing for 30 seconds. Towards the end of 30 seconds period inject 0.1 ml of acetylcholine solution into the inner organ tube and record the tracing for

90 seconds. Finally after 90 seconds turn off the kymograph and give 3 - 4 washings of rectus muscle with tyrode solution.

9. Inject 0.1 ml of acetylcholine solution into the inner organ tube once again and trace the response for 90 seconds.

10. If two equipotent responses are observed with similar doses of acetylcholine, then trace the responses of ach by using high doses (0.2, 0.4, 0.8 and 1 ml) as shown in Fig. 12.1.

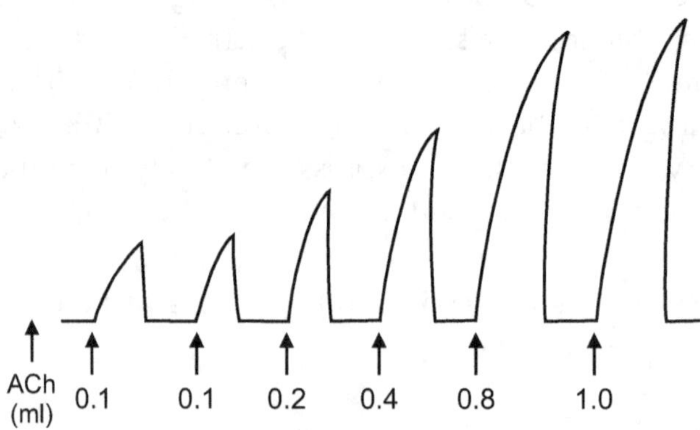

Fig. 12.1: Dose response curve of acetylcholine

11. After fixing the graph measure the height of contraction of the response produced by each dose of ACh and also find out the dose which produces maximal response.

OBSERVATIONS:

Sr. No.	Dose of acetylcholine in ml	Log dose of Acetylcholine	Height of contraction (Response) in mm	% Response
1	0.1			
2	0.2			
3	0.4			
4	0.6			
5	0.8			
6	1.0			

12. Plot a graph showing dose of ACh on X-axis and response on Y-axis.

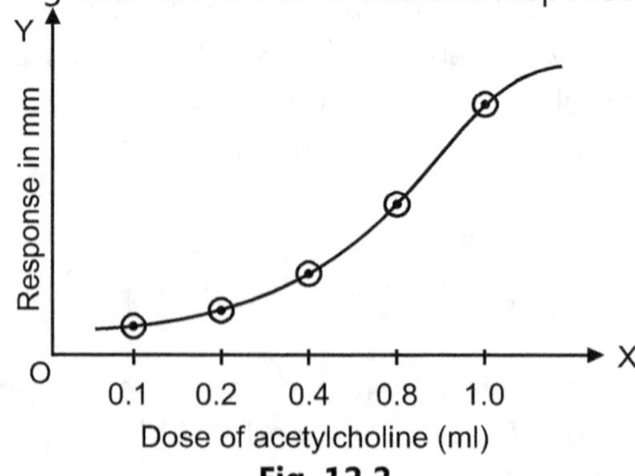

Fig. 12.2

13. Plot the DRC on semilog graph paper taking log dose of agonist on X- axis and % response on Y-axis.

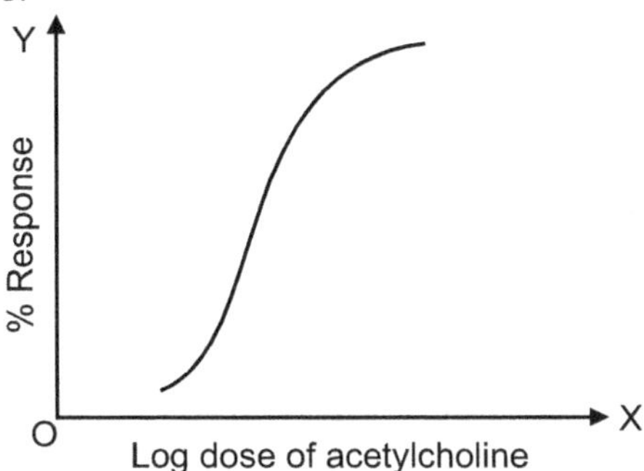

Fig. 12.3

14. Plot a third graph showing log molar conc. of ACh on X-axis and % response on Y-axis.

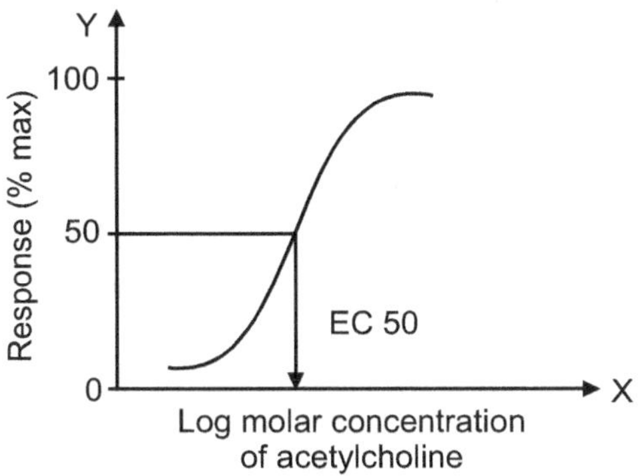

Fig. 12.4

15. With the help of graph find out the EC50 value and pD_2 value.

For example,

If the EC50 = $M \times 10^{-n}$ = 9.5×10^{-7}

Then, pD_2 = n – log m = 7 – log 9.5 = 7 – 0.98 = 6.03.

Therefore one can define pD_2 value as the negative log of molar concentration of drug exhibiting half of the maximum response.

pD_2 value gives information about affinity of a drug for a particular receptor.

Suppose,

Drug A has pD_2 value = 5.02

Drug B has pD_2 value = 6.03

Drug C has pD_2 value = 7

Then this indicates that drug C is most potent drug.

VIVA VOCE QUESTIONS

1. Explain pD_2 value.

Ans. The EC50 value describes relative potency of the drugs. Lower the EC50 value, more potent is the drug. Sometimes the same is indicated as pD_2 value which is defined as negative log of molar concentration of the drug producing 50% of maximal response. If pD_2 value is high, then the potency is also high. In calculating the pD_2 value, the % of the maximum response produced by each dose (concentration) is plotted against log molar concentration of the drug and the concentration producing 50% response is read as pD_2 value. The EC50 or pD_2 values are used to express the affinity of a drug. Both the values can be interconvertible employing a simple equation i.e. if EC50 expressed as $(m \times 10^{-n})$, then $pD_2 = n - \log m$.

Dose ratio (EC50) is calculated by comparing the doses of ACh, needed to produce 50% response in presence and absence of drug.

2. Define pD_2 value.

Ans. pD_2 value is defined as negative log of molar concentration of the drug producing 50% of maximum response. If pD_2 value is high, then the potency is also high.

3. How will you calculate dose ratio ?

Ans. Dose ratio (EC50) is calculated by comparing the doses of ACh, needed to produce 50% response in the presence and absence of drug.

4. pD_2 value gives information about ......

Ans. pD_2 value gives information about affinity of a drug for a particular receptor.

5. How much time is needed for tissue stabilization ?

Ans. 30 minutes are needed for tissues stabilization.

MULTIPLE CHOICE QUESTIONS (MCQ'S)

1. Select the PSS used in this experiment.
  (a) Frog ringer solution
  (b) Tyrode solution
  (c) De Jalon solution
  (d) Krebs solution

2. Select the correct dose of acetylcholine :
  (a) 1 mg/ml
  (b) 2 mg/ml
  (c) 3 mg/ml
  (d) 4 mg/ml

3. Which part of guinea pig is used for study?
  (a) Jejunum
  (b) Deuodenum
  (c) Ileum
  (d) Rectus abdominis muscle

4. Tension on the frog rectus abdominis muscle is :
  (a) 500 mg
  (b) 1 gm
  (c) 1.5 gm
  (d) None of above

5. The EC50 value describes relative potency of the drugs. Lower the EC50 value, more potent is the drug.
  (a) True
  (b) False

Answers :

1. (b)	2. (a)	3. (c)	4. (a)	5. (a)

***

Experiment No. 13

Aim: Effect of spasmogens and spasmolytics using rabbit jejunum.

INTRODUCTION:

Spasmogens: It is a substance which induces spasms or a substance which can produce contraction of smooth muscle such as histamine, serotonin, bradykinin etc.

Spasmolytics: These are also called as antispasmodic. These are accountable for smooth muscle relaxation. An antispasmodic is pharmaceutical drug that suppresses muscle spasms.

PRINCIPLE:

Rabbit intestine is a smooth muscle which shows regular pendular movement (i.e. nonstop contraction and relaxation). Therefore, for studying effect of drugs on intestinal movement, rabbit intestine is an ideal preparation. Rabbit intestine is supplied by ANS. Rabbit intestine contains muscarinic receptors and adrenergic receptors. Muscarinic receptors agonist like acetylcholine produces contraction of rabbit intestine and physostigmine increases the spasm and pendular movements. The above muscarinic actions and effects are obstructed by muscarinic blockers.

Adrenaline acts on alpha and beta receptors and exhibits inhibitory effect on pendular movements. The adrenaline action is inhibited by adrenoreceptor blockers like alpha receptor blockers and beta receptor blockers.

REQUIREMENTS:

Equipments and Apparatus: Kymograph, student thermostatic organ bath, aerator, frontal writing lever, haemostatic forceps, mariotte bottle, rubber tubes, tuberculine syringe, suturing needle, scissor, etc.

Animal: Rabbit.

Tissue: Jejunum.

Drugs: Acetylcholine (20 µg /ml)

Physostigmine (10 µg /ml)

Atropine (4 µg/ml)

Adrenaline (20 µg /ml)

Propranolol (100 µg /ml)

PSS: Tyrode solution.

Tension on the tissue: 500 mg

Magnification: 10 times.

PROCEDURE:

1. Fast a rabbit for 12 hours period.
2. Set up the assembly for rabbit jejunum experiment.
3. Balance a frontal writing lever using plasticine and apply 500 mg tension.
4. Fill the outer jacket of student organ tube by using water.

5.   Set the thermostat of the student organ bath at 37°C and put the switch on.
6.   Fill the mariotte bottle with tyrode solution and control stream of tyrode solution to the inner organ tube using haemostatic forceps.
7.   When the temperature of the tyrode solution reaches 37°C, kill a rabbit by giving a blow on its head and cutting the carotid artery.
8.   Open the abdominal cavity and identify the intestine.
9.   Remove a length of jejunum and place it in a petridish which contains tyrode solution at 37°C and trim away the mesentery.
10.   Cut a portion of jejunum (approximately 2 - 3 cm) and using surgical suturing needle tie a thread at each end, taking care to see that the lumen of the jejunum remained open.
11.   Tie one end of the thread to the hook of the aeration tube and the other to a frontal writing lever.
12.   Tissue is stabilizing for 30 minutes.
13.   Aerate the rabbit jejunum in the inner organ tube with oxygen (95 %) and carbon dioxide (5 %) (Carbogen) mixture.
14.   Record the normal pendular movement of rabbit jejunum on the drum for 30 seconds. At the end of 30 seconds add 0.1 ml of acetylcholine into the inner organ tube and record the Spasmogenic effect of the drug for 30 seconds. After recording the response for 30 seconds turn off kymograph. Immediately open the outlet of the inner organ tube and remove the tyrode solution present in inner organ bath.
15.   Again fill the organ tube with fresh solution of tyrode and keep it for 60 seconds. Repeat the washing procedure 3 – 4 times or till the writing point of the frontal lever comes to the normal pendular movement base line.
16.   Trace the response of 0.1 ml physostigmine solution. Give 3 - 4 washings for recovery.
17.   Trace the response of 0.1 ml adrenaline solution. Give 3 - 4 washings for recovery.
18.   Add 0.1 ml of atropine sulphate solution into the inner organ tube, allow it to act for 60 seconds. Then trace the response of ACh in atropine sulphate presence. Give 3 - 4 washings for recovery.
19.   Add 0.1 ml of atropine sulphate solution into the inner organ tube, allow it to act for 60 seconds. Then trace the response of physostigmine solution in the presence of atropine sulphate. Give 3 - 4 washings for recovery.
20.   Add 0.1 ml of propranolol solution into the inner organ bath, allow it to act for 60 seconds. Then record the response of adrenaline solution in the presence of propranolol. Give 3 - 4 washings for recovery.

DISCUSSION:

Acetylcholine produced contraction of the rabbit jejunum. Atropine sulphate is a muscarinic receptors blocker; therefore it reduced the spasmogenic effect caused by acetylcholine. Physostigmine also produced mild spasmogenic effect and increased the peristaltic movement of the jejunum. Atropine sulphate blocks the effect of physostigmine.

VIVA VOCE QUESTIONS

1. Define spasmogens and spasmolytics.

Ans. **Spasmogens:** A substance which induces spasms or a substance that can produce contraction of smooth muscles such as histamine, serotonin, bradykinin etc. is called spasmogens.

Spasmolytics: These are called as antispasmodic. These are responsible for relaxation of smooth muscles. An antispasmodic is a pharmaceutical drug which suppresses muscle spasms.

2. Give the principle in study of spasmogens and spasmolytics using rabbit jejunum.

Ans. Rabbit intestine is a smooth muscle which shows regular pendular movement (i.e. nonstop contraction and relaxation). Therefore, for studying effect of drugs on intestinal movement, rabbit intestine is an ideal preparation. Rabbit intestine is supplied by ANS. Rabbit intestine contains muscarinic receptors and adrenergic receptors. Muscarinic receptors agonist like acetylcholine produces contraction of rabbit intestine and physostigmine increases the spasm and pendular movements. The above muscarinic actions and effects are obstructed by muscarinic blockers.

Adrenaline acts on alpha and beta receptors and exhibits inhibitory effect on pendular movements. The adrenaline action is inhibited by adrenoreceptor blockers like alpha receptor blockers and beta receptor blockers.

3. Explain MOA of physostigmine.

Ans. Physostigmine represses acetylcholinesterase, the chemical in charge of the breakdown of utilized acetylcholine. By meddling with the digestion of acetylcholine, physostigmine in a roundabout way invigorates both nicotinic and muscarinic receptors because of the considerable increment in accessible acetylcholine at the neural connection.

4. Write uses of propranolol.

Ans. Propranolol is a beta blocker used to treat high BP, arrhythmia. It is used after a heart attack. Also useful for prevention of migraine headaches and chest pain (angina). Lowering high blood pressure helps prevent strokes, heart attacks, and kidney problems.

5. Write uses of atropine sulphate.

Ans. Atropine sulphate is anticholinergic drug and is used to treat certain eye conditions (e.g., uveitis). Atropine widens (dilating) the pupil of the eye etc.

MULTIPLE CHOICE QUESTIONS (MCQ'S)

1. **Which animal is used for spasmogens and spasmolytics study?**

   (a) Guinea pig   (b) Frog

   (c) Rabbit   (d) Rat

2. **Which part of animal is used for spasmogens and spasmolytics study?**

   (a) Stomach   (b) Duodenum

   (c) Jejunum   (d) Ileum

3. **Which PSS is used for spasmogens and spasmolytics study on rabbit jejunum?**

   (a) Ringer solution   (b) Krebs solution

   (c) De Jalon solution   (d) Tyrode solution

4. **Select correct example of spasmogenic :**

   (a) Acetylcholine   (b) Histamine

   (c) $BaCl_2$ (d) All of these

5. **Atropine sulphate is a muscarinic receptors blocker; therefore it reduces the spasmogenic effect caused by acetylcholine.**

   (a) True   (b) False

Answers :

1. (c)	2. (c)	3. (d)	4. (d)	5. (a)

***

Experiment No. 14

Aim: To study anti-inflammatory activity of drugs using carrageenan induced paw edema model.

INTRODUCTION:

Inflammation:

It is reply of immune system to foreign organism or antigenic substance. It is characterized by edema, erythema, swelling, pain, tenderness and burning sensation.

Signs of Inflammation: The five classical signs of inflammation are heat, pain, redness, swelling, and loss of function (Latin: calor, dolor, rubor, tumor, and functio laesa).

Classification of Inflammation: Inflammation can be classified as either acute or chronic.

1. Acute inflammation
2. Chronic inflammation

Phases of Inflammation:

- **Acute:** Vasodilation and increase capillary permeability.
- **Delayed:** Infiltration of leukocytes and phagocyte cells.
- **Chronic proliferative:** Tissue degeneration and fibrosis.

Mediators of Inflammation:

- Bradykinin
- Leukocytes
- Lysosome granules
- Histamine
- T-cells, NK cells
- Leukotriene
- Interleukins
- Prostaglandins

Anti-inflammatory Drugs:

1. **Steroidal:** Example: Corticosteroids etc.
2. **Non-steroidal Anti-inflammatory Drugs (NSAID):** Examples: Acetyl salicylic acid, indomethacin, ibuprofen, etc.

Indomethacin is a NSAID used to reduce fever, pain, stiffness, and swelling. It acts by preventing the production of prostaglandin molecules responsible for above symptoms.

PRINCIPLE:

The provocative response is promptly created in rodents as paw edema with the assistance of irritants. Substances, for example, carrageenan, formalin, bradykinin, histamine, 5-hydroxytryptamine, mustard or egg white when infused in the dorsum of the foot of rodents, they deliver intense paw edema inside a couple of minutes of the infusion.

Carrageenan is a sulphated polysaccharide acquired from ocean weed and by causing the arrival of histamine, 5-HT, bradykinin and prostaglandins it produces aggravation and edema.

This strategy depends on the capacity of calming specialists to restrain the edema delivered in the rear paw of the rodent after infusion of carrageenan. The volume of infused paw is estimated when the utilization of the aggravations. The paw volume of treated creatures is contrasted and controlled. Plethysmograph is utilized to measure the paw volume.

Plethysmograph: It is a basic mechanical assembly containing mercury. The mercury uprooting due to plunging of the paw can be straightforwardly persued from the scale appended to the mercury section or modifying the mercury level in the arm B to the first level by moving of B up/down and taking note of the volume required to get the level of both the arms equivalent.

REQUIREMENTS:

Equipments and Apparatus: Plethysmograph, vernier calipers, syringes, oral feeding tube, etc.

Animal: Rat (150-200 g).

Drugs and Solutions:

1. Carrageenan (prepare 1% w/v solution and inject 0.1 ml into planter region).
2. Indomethacin (20 mg/kg, s.c., stock solution - 4 mg/ml of the drug and inject 0.5 ml/100 g of the body weight of the rat).
3. Normal saline solution.

PROCEDURE:

1. Weigh the animals of either sex and number them.
2. Make the mark on both the rear paws (right and left) just past tibio-tarsal intersection, with the goal that each time the paw is plunged in the mercury segment upto the fixed imprint to guarantee steady paw volume.
3. Note the underlying paw volume (right and left) of each animal by mercury displacement strategy.
4. Divide the rats into two groups each including in any event four animals.
5. To one group administer saline and to the subsequent group administer indomethacin subcutaneously.
6. After 30 minutes infuse 0.1 ml of 1% w/v carrageenan in the planter area of the left paw of control just as indomethacin treated group. The right paw will serve as reference non-inflamed paw for comparison.
7. Note the paw volume of both the legs of control and indomethacin treated rats at 15, 30, 60, and 120 minutes after carrageenan challenge.
8. Calculate the % difference in the right and left paw volumes of each animal of control and indomethacin treated group.
9. Compare the mean % change in the paw volume in control and drug treated animals and express as % edema inhibition by the indomethacin.

OBSERVATIONS:

Table 14.1: Anti-inflammatory activity of indomethacin by using carrageenan induced paw edema in rats

Sr. No.	Body wt. (g)	Treatment	Dose (mg/kg)	Paw volume (ml) as measured by mercury displacement at									
				0 (min)		15 (min)		30 (min)		60 (min)		120 (min)	
				R	L	R	L	R	L	R	L	R	L
1	150	Control											
2	155	Control											
3	160	Control											
4	165	Control											
			Mean										
			% difference in R and L										
1	150	Indomethacin	20, s.c.										
2	155	Indom.											
3	160	Indom.											
4	165	Indom.											
			Mean										
			% difference in R and L										

R = Right paw, *L = Inject 0.1 ml of 1% w/v carrageenan 30 minutes after indomethacin to the left paw by sub planter route.

Calculate % edema inhibition at different time intervals.

DISCUSSION:

Indomethacin showed anti-inflammatory action against carrageenan-induced paw edema.

Inflammation is clinically characterized as rubor (redness), calor (heat), tumor (swelling) and dolor (pain). It has three phases. The first phase is due to increase in vascular permeability resulting in exudation of fluid from the blood into the interstitial space. The second phase involves infiltration of leukocytes from the blood into the tissue and third phase is granuloma formation.

Indomethacin is powerful anti-inflammatory agent with analgesic and antipyretic properties. Indomethacin inhibits production of eicosanoids like prostacyclin, thromboxane and prostaglandins by inhibition of cyclo-oxygenase (COX) and thereby reduces edema in this model.

Paw edema is the method used for testing acute inflammation. Among other methods of screening, this is simple and most commonly used technique. It is rapid as well as reproducible method. It is used to estimate duration of action and potency of corticosteroids after systematic as well as local application.

VIVA VOCE QUESTIONS

1. Define Inflammation and write its phases.

Ans. Inflammation is reply of immune system to foreign organism or antigenic substance. It is characterized by edema, erythema, swelling, and pain or tenderness.

Phases of inflammation:

Acute: Vasodilation and increased capillary permeability.

Delayed: Infiltration of leukocytes and phagocyte cells.

Chronic proliferative: Tissue degeneration and fibrosis.

2. Enlist mediators in inflammation.

Ans.
- Bradykinin
- Histamine
- Interleukins
- Leukocytes
- T-cells, NK cells
- Prostaglandins
- Lysosome granules
- Leukotriene

3. Explain Plethysmograph.

Ans. It is a basic mechanical assembly containing mercury. The mercury uprooting due to plunging of the paw can be straightforwardly persued from the scale appended to the mercury section or modifying the mercury level in the arm B to the first level by moving of B up/down and taking note of the volume required to get the level of both the arms equivalent.

4. Explain MOA of Indomethacin.

Ans. Indomethacin is a NSAID used to reduce fever, pain, stiffness, and swelling. It acts by preventing the production of prostaglandins molecules responsible for above symptoms.

5. Give the principle in anti-inflammatory activity of drugs using carrageenan induced paw edema model.

Ans. The provocative response is promptly created in rodents as paw edema with the assistance of aggravations. Substances, for example, carrageenan, formalin, bradykinin, histamine, 5-hydroxytryptamine, mustard or egg white when infused in the dorsum of the foot of rodents, they deliver intense paw edema inside a couple of minutes of the infusion.

Carrageenan is a sulphated polysaccharide acquired from ocean weed and by causing the arrival of histamine, 5-HT, bradykinin and prostaglandins, it produces aggravation and edema.

This strategy depends on the capacity of calming specialists to restrain the edema delivered in the rear paw of the rodent after infusion of carrageenan. The volume of infused paw is estimated when the utilization of the aggravations. The paw volume of treated creatures is contrasted and controlled. Plethysmograph is utilized to measure the paw volume.

MULTIPLE CHOICE QUESTIONS (MCQ'S)

1. **Which animal is used for anti-inflammatory activity?**
   - (a) Frog
   - (b) Rabbit
   - (c) Rat
   - (d) Guinea pig

2. **Select correct anti-inflammatory agent :**
   - (a) Cisplatin
   - (b) Indomethacin
   - (c) Chloroquine
   - (d) Tetracycline

3. **Inflammatory response is produced by :**
   - (a) Carrageenan
   - (b) Bradykinin
   - (c) Formalin
   - (d) All of these

4. **Which apparatus is used to measure the paw volume?**
   - (a) Haemocytometer
   - (b) Sphygmomanometer
   - (c) Plethysmograph
   - (d) None of these

5. **Carrageenan is a sulphated polysaccharide obtained from sea weed and by causing the release of histamine, 5-HT, bradykinin and prostaglandins it produces inflammation and edema.**
   - (a) True
   - (b) False

Answers:

1. (c)	2. (b)	3. (d)	4. (c)	5. (a)

***

Experiment No. 15

Aim: To study analgesic activity of drug using central and peripheral methods.

1. CENTRAL METHOD:

Objective: Analgesic activity of morphine in mice using hot plate method (Central method).

INTRODUCTION:

Absence of pain is characterized as a condition of diminished attention to pain and analgesics are the substances which diminish sensation of pain by increasing threshold to the painful stimuli. The regularly utilized analgesics are headache medicine, paracetamol (non-opiate) and morphine (opiate) and so forth.

Agonizing response in exploratory creatures can be delivered by applying toxic (upsetting) improvements, for example,

1.   Thermal (Radiant heat is source of pain),

2.   Chemicals (acetic acid and bradykinin) and

3.   Physical pressure (by compression of tail).

Morphine:

Morphine is a pain medication of the opiate family which is obtained naturally from various plants. It works on the central nervous system (CNS) to diminish the pain sensation. It is used for both acute pain and chronic pain. It is regularly utilized for pain from myocardial infarction and during labor. It is administered orally by injection into the muscle and under the skin, intravenously, injection into the space around the spinal cord, or rectally. Maximum result is attained within 20 minutes when given intravenously and after 60 minutes when given by mouth.

Side effects include a diminished respiratory values and low blood pressure. Morphine is responsible for addiction and abuse. If amount is decreased after long-term use, withdrawal may occur. Common SE is drowsiness, vomiting, and constipation. Caution is advised when used during pregnancy or breast feeding, as morphine will affect the baby.

MOA of Morphine: The exact component of the pain relieving activity of morphine is obscure. Be that as it may, explicit CNS sedative receptors have been distinguished and likely assume a job in the statement of pain relieving impacts. Morphine first follows up on the mu-narcotic receptors. The system of respiratory discouragement includes a decrease in the responsiveness of the cerebrum stem respiratory focuses to increments in carbon dioxide pressure and to electrical incitement. It has been demonstrated that morphine ties to and hinders GABA inhibitory interneurons. These interneurons ordinarily repress the pain restraint pathway. In this way, without the inhibitory sign, pain regulation can continue downstream.

PRINCIPLE:

Animal is presenting to the toxic improvement. In this strategy warmth is utilized as a wellspring of torment and the time taken to deliver reaction like paw - licking and hopping are recorded. Animals are independently set on a hot plate kept up at consistent temperature (55°C) and the response of animals; for example, paw licking or jumping reaction is taken as the end point.

Hind paw licking is shown within 4-6 seconds and following 2-3 seconds jumping may begin. Watch these reactions while organization of medication. Analgesics increase the response time.

REQUIREMENTS:

Animals: Mice (20 – 25 g).

Drugs: Morphine sulphate (5 mg/kg, sc, stock solution - 0.5 mg/ml and inject 1 ml/100 g of body weight of mice).

Equipment: Eddy's hot plate.

PROCEDURE:

1. Weigh the animals of any sex and number them.

2. Take the basal response time by watching rear paw licking or bouncing reaction (whichever shows up first) in mice when put on the hot plate kept up at steady temperature (55°C).

3. Normally the mice shows such reaction in 6 - 8 seconds. A cut off time of 15 seconds is seen to evade harm to the paws.

4. Inject morphine to the mice and note the response time of mice on the hot plate at 15, 30, 60 and 120 minutes after the administration of drug.

5. As the response time increases with morphine 15 seconds are taken as most extreme absence of pain and the mice are expelled from the hot plate to avoid damage to the paws.

6. Calculate the percent expansion in response time at each time interim.

OBSERVATIONS:

Table 15.1: Analgesic activity of morphine using tail flick method

Sr. No.	Body weight	Basal reaction time (sec) (Before Morphine admin)		Reaction time (sec) (After Morphine administration)	
		Paw licking	Jump response	Paw licking	Jump response
1					
2					
3					
4					
5					

Dose: 5 mg/kg morphine is administered, subcutaneously.

* A cut off time of 15 seconds is taken as greatest pain relieving reaction to avoid damage to the paws.

2. PERIPHERAL METHOD:

Objective: Analgesic activity of morphine against acetic acid induced writhing in mice (Peripheral method).

INTRODUCTION:

Writhing Response: It is a response or painful reaction shown by an animal following administration of certain chemicals. Writhing response includes abdomen constriction, twisting of trunk and the expansion of hind legs.

PRINCIPLE:

Writhing provoked by acetic acid is painful response which can be described by recognizable signs like narrowing of mid-region, turning of trunk and the expansion of rear legs. Excruciating response in animals might be delivered by synthetic compounds, for example, phenylquinone, bradykinin and so on, which are portrayed as a writhing reaction. Analgesics both narcotics and non-narcotics type, inhibit writhing response.

REQUIREMENTS:

Animals: Mice (25 – 30 g).

Apparatus: Syringe, glass jar, etc.

Drugs and Solutions:

1. Morphine sul. (5 mg/kg, sc, stock solution - 0.5 mg/ml and administer 1 ml/100 g of body weight of animal).
2. Acetic acid 1% v/v (Inject 1 ml/100 g of body weight of the animals).
3. Normal Saline (0.9%).

PROCEDURE:

1. Weigh the animals of any sex and number them.
2. Separate mice into 2 groups, consisting of 5 animals. Administer appropriate volume of solution of acetic acid to first group (control group).
3. Place them exclusively under glass container for observation.
4. Note the beginning of wriths. Record the quantity of contraction of abdomen, twisting of trunk and rear limb extension.
5. Inject morphine to the second group of animals. 15 minutes later, administer acetic acid solution of these animals.
6. Note the beginning and seriousness of writhing reaction as contraction of abdomen, trunk twist reaction and expansion of rear legs and the quantity of mice indicating such reaction during a time of 10 minutes.
7. Calculate the mean writhing reaction in control and morphine treated groups. Note the inhibition of pain response by morphine.

OBSERVATIONS:

Table 15.2: Analgesic activity of morphine in mice using hot plate method

Sr. No.	Body weight (gm)	Treatment	No. of writhing (10 min)	Responders (n/n)
1				
2				
3		Control (Acetic acid)		
4				
5				
		Mean		
1				
2				
3		Morphine + Acetic acid		
4				
5				
		Mean		

VIVA VOCE QUESTIONS

1. Define analgesia.

Ans. Absence of pain is characterized as a condition of diminished attention to pain and analgesics are the substances which diminish sensation of pain by increasing threshold to the painful stimuli.

2. Painful reactions in animals are produced by which techniques?

Ans. Painful reactions in experimental animals can be produced by applying noxious (unpleasant) stimuli such as: (a) Thermal, (b) Chemicals and (c) Physical pressure.

3. Explain the MOA of morphine.

Ans. The exact component of the pain relieving activity of morphine is obscure. Be that as it may, explicit CNS sedative receptors have been distinguished and likely assume a job in the statement of pain relieving impacts. Morphine first follows up on the mu-narcotic receptors. The system of respiratory discouragement includes a decrease in the responsiveness of the cerebrum stem respiratory focuses to increments in carbon dioxide pressure and to electrical incitement. It has been demonstrated that morphine ties to and hinders GABA inhibitory interneurons. These interneurons ordinarily repress the pain restraint pathway. In this way, without the inhibitory sign, pain regulation can continue downstream.

4. Write symptoms of writhing response.

Ans. Writhing response includes abdomen constriction, trunk twisting and the extension of rear legs.

5. Which apparatus is used for measuring central analgesics activity?

Ans. For measuring the central analgesic activity Eddy's Hot plate is used.

MULTIPLE CHOICE QUESTIONS (MCQ'S)

1. Which animal is used for analgesic activity?

(a) Frog   (b) Mice

(c) Rabbit   (d) Guinea pig

2. Select correct dose of morphine in central analgesic activity :

(a) 1 mg/kg   (b) 2 mg/kg

(c) 3 mg/kg   (d) 5 mg/kg

3. **Temperature of Eddy's hot plate maintained at :**

   (a) 45°C

   (b) 50°C

   (c) 55°C

   (d) 60°C

4. **Writhing response induced by :**

   (a) Acetic acid

   (b) Bradykinin

   (c) Phenylquinone

   (d) All of these

5. **Analgesics, both narcotics and non-narcotics type, inhibit writhing response.**

   (a) True

   (b) False

Answers:

1. (b)	2. (d)	3. (c)	4. (d)	5. (a)

✷✷✷

BIBLIOGRAPHY

- A Handbook of Experiments in Preclinical Pharmacology, Sanjay B. Kasture, 1st edition, 2010, Career Publication, Nashik.
- Drug Discovery and Evaluation: Pharmacological Assay, H. G. Vogel and W. H. Vogel, 3rd edition, 2008, Springer - Verlag Berlin Heidelberg New York.
- Experimental Pharmacology, K. K. Pillai, 1st edition, 2010, CBS Publisher and Distributor Pvt. Ltd, New Delhi.
- Fundamentals of Experimental Pharmacology, M. N. Ghosh, 4th edition, 2008, Hilton and Company, Kolkata.
- Gerald Poch, et al, Construction of antagonist dose-response curves for estimation of pA2-values by Schild-plot analysis and detection of allosteric interactions, Br. J. Pharmacology (1992), 106, 710 - 716.
- Handbook of Experimental Pharmacology by S. K. Kulkarni, 4th edition, 2012, Vallabh Prakashan, New Delhi.
- http://www.biology-pages.info/A/AnimalHearts.html
- http://www.geneticalliance.org/programs/biotrust/nets/content/in_vitro
- http://www.microbiologynotes.com/detailed-structure-of-frogs-heart/
- https://en.wikipedia.org/wiki/In_vitro
- https://www.petcoach.co/article/hypertension-high-blood-pressure-in-dogs-and-cats/
- https://www.thesprucepets.com/normal-temperature-heart-rates-in-dogs-4143223
- Laboratory Manual, Experimental Pharmacology, Dr. Huda Kafeel, 2014,113 – 116.
- Laboratory Procedure Manual Ms. Love Julian, Coulston Foundation, Alamogordo, New Mexico, 1999–2000.
- Marcio A. F. et al, Cross-Talk Between AT1 and AT2 Angiotensin Receptors in Rat Anococcygeus Smooth Muscle, The Journal of Pharmacology and Experimental Therapeutics , by The American Society for Pharmacology and Experimental Therapeutics, Vol. 303, No. 1, 333–339, 2002.
- Practicals in Pharmacology, Dr. R. K. Goyal, 11th edition, 2013 – 14, B. S. Shah Prakashan, Ahmedabad.
- R. J. Tallarida et al., pA2 Analysis I: Schild Plot, Manual of Pharmacologic Calculations, Springer -Verlag New York Inc. 1987, 53 – 54.
- Slobodan M. et al, Schild's Equation and the Best Estimate of pA2 Value and Dissociation Constant of an Antagonist, Croatian Medical Journal, March 1999, Volume 40, Number 1.
- Sunil J Panuganti, Principles Involved in Bioassay by Different Methods: A Mini-Review, Principles Involved in Bioassay by different Methods: A Mini-Review, Volume 3, Issue 2, April - June, 2015, 1 – 18.

****